# THE
# KOREAN
# SKINCARE
# BIBLE

한국스킨케어의 예술

**MiiN**

# THE
# KOREAN
# SKINCARE
# BIBLE

한국스킨케어의 예술

**LILIN YANG | LEAH GANSE | SARA JIMÉNEZ**

An Hachette UK Company
www.hachette.co.uk

First published in Great Britain in 2019 by Cassell,
an imprint of Octopus Publishing Group Ltd,
Carmelite House,
50 Victoria Embankment,
London EC4Y 0DZ
www.octopusbooks.co.uk
www.octopusbooksusa.com

© MiiN Cosmetics, S.L., 2018
Lilin Yang, Leah Ganse and Sara Jiménez (text)
Esther Sandoval (make-up chapter)

Originally published in Spain as: *El arte coreano del cuidado de la piel* by MiiN Cosmetics, S.L.
© Editorial Planeta, S.A., 2018
Zenith is an imprint of Editorial Planeta, S.A
Avda. Diagonal 662-664, 08034 Barcelona (Spain)

© Inner design: Georgina Gerónimo

Text copyright © Octopus Publishing Group 2019
Design and layout copyright © Octopus Publishing Group 2019

Distributed in the US by Hachette Book Group,
1290 Avenue of the Americas,
4th and 5th Floors, New York, NY 10104

Distributed in Canada by Canadian Manda Group,
664 Annette St., Toronto,
Ontario, Canada M6S 2C8

ISBN 978-1-78840-166-1

A CIP catalogue record for this book is available from the British Library.

Printed and bound in China.

10 9 8 7 6 5 4 3

Commissioning Editor: Romilly Morgan
Editorial Assistant: Mireille Harper
Translator: Jordan Lancaster
Copy Editor: Patricia Burgess
Proofreader: Clare Churly
Art Director: Juliette Norsworthy
Additional Illustrations: Claire Huntley
Production Controller: Sarah Kulasek-Boyd

# CONTENTS

# INTRODUCTION

You've probably heard about Korean cosmetics, but you might not know how they arrived in Europe through MiiN.

I've been living in Spain for more than ten years, and even though my lifestyle has changed a great deal since I arrived from Asia, THERE'S ONE THING I DIDN'T WANT TO LEAVE BEHIND: MY SKINCARE ROUTINE.

My mother has always been my inspiration. Without a doubt, she is the reason I am interested in the world of cosmetics and personal care. I remember how she would sit in front of the mirror with dozens of different products. My father and I didn't really understand what she was doing, but for her those moments alone were practically sacred. The fact that she took such pleasure in her beauty ritual drew me to her side to watch how she did it.

Over time, she introduced me to the marvellous world of beauty. When I was 14 years old and still living in China, my mother gave me my first set of skincare products. By the time I was 16, I was purchasing products with my own money. My choices were basic: a moisturiser and a cleanser. From that day on, I have used beauty products every day of my life.

When I moved to Spain, I lived in Madrid for a time, but I never stopped visiting Asia – places such as Hong Kong, Seoul and Taiwan. On these trips, I would fill my suitcase with new cosmetics and treatments because in Europe I was unable to find everything I needed, and the latest trends were always 'made in South Korea'.

THE MIIN CONCEPT BEGAN WITH A PERSONAL NEED BECAUSE TRAVELLING THOUSANDS OF MILES TO PURCHASE COSMETICS WASN'T AN IDEAL SOLUTION. I remember that on one of my visits I had to queue to enter a Korean cosmetic shop offering one of the most famous brands. Queuing to enter a shop? How bizarre! It seemed like every Asian woman was craving these products yet they were still unknown in Europe, and I kept asking myself why...

This led me to formulate a plan to introduce my favourite brands to Europe. In this way, it would be easier for me to buy them and it would also allow European women to discover their excellent properties. The venture involved a great deal of time and effort, particularly at the beginning, as I was still studying at university, but I loved every minute of it, and still do.

IN 2014, WE OPENED OUR FIRST SHOP IN THE EIXAMPLE AREA OF BARCELONA. It wasn't easy to start with. Cosmetics play a very important role in people's lives, because they use the products every day in direct contact with their skin, they need to trust the brands they use.

How could it be that the best cosmetics in the world came from a country so far away? During the first few months, the MiiN team was still very small and focused on sharing the word about the virtues and special qualities of Korean cosmetics. People soon began to look for information on the products by themselves and would come to the shop with specific queries.

So great was the demand that the shop in Barcelona became the starting point for something much larger: expansion throughout Europe. Our first step was to open an online shop in five languages. After that, we opened shops in various locations: Madrid in the summer of 2015, Munich in 2016, then Paris and Milan, two incredible cities where we hope that Korean cosmetics will make their mark. Our shops are small and welcoming; this is our hallmark. We try to address the smallest of details, and of course we pay special attention to the selection of products.

WHY ARE WE CALLED MIIN COSMETICS?
MIIN ACTUALLY REPRESENTS TWO KOREAN WORDS, *MI* AND *IN*, WHICH MEAN 'BEAUTIFUL WOMAN'. THE COMPANY LOGO IS BASED ON THE KOREAN SPELLING OF THESE WORDS AND IS A MIXTURE OF TRADITIONAL AND MODERN LETTERING, WHICH ADDS A TOUCH OF *KAWAII* (CUTENESS) TO THE FACE.

By moving into the international sphere, we have been able to observe cultural differences in client choices, which we enjoy. We learn something new every day. Although our story is short, we hope it will have a very long future. So, if you want to enter the fascinating world of Korean cosmetics, all you have to do is keep reading.

FOR MIIN, BEAUTY IS ABOUT WELLNESS AND CARING FOR YOURSELF. WHAT WE LOVE MOST ABOUT THE KOREAN BEAUTY ROUTINE IS THAT IT ALLOWS YOU TO TAKE A FEW MINUTES EVERY DAY JUST FOR YOU TO FEEL AND BE BETTER. BEAUTY IS A RITUAL. It's not just about looking good; it's also about caring for yourself.

### WHY WRITE A BOOK ABOUT KOREAN COSMETICS?

The MiiN team has always known that Korean cosmetics are more than just a passing trend. However, sharing the benefits of them with the general public required us to amass a great deal of information. We can't sell something that people don't trust and believe in. Therefore, it's very important that we teach and demonstrate the strengths and innovations of South Korean cosmetics. Over the past four years, we have answered and resolved literally thousands of queries. It's no wonder, then, that compiling them in a book seemed the obvious way to bring all that information together and satisfy our clients' curiosity. How did Korean cosmetics begin? Why are they so esteemed? What products should I use? Where can I find the ten steps of the Korean beauty routine? All the answers are within this book.

WELCOME TO *THE KOREAN SKINCARE BIBLE*.

LILIN YANG
Founder of MiiN Cosmetics

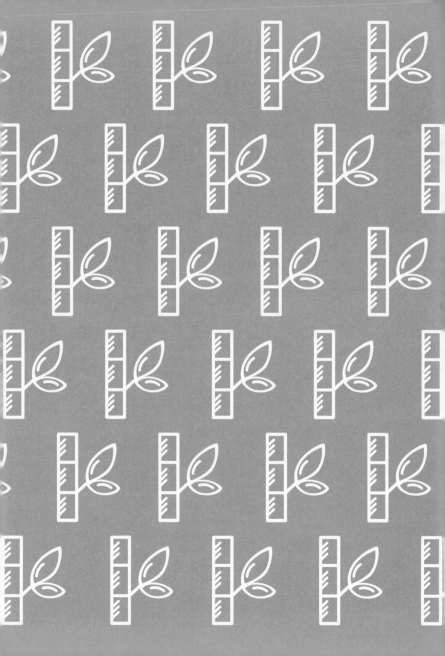

# 01

---

## THE HISTORY OF KOREAN BEAUTY

한국 스킨케어의 역사

---

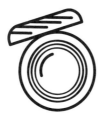

WHAT WE KNOW NOW ABOUT KOREAN COSMETICS IS ONLY THE TIP OF THE ICEBERG. Their successful history goes back many centuries and reads like a fairy tale.

Once upon a time, so long ago that the exact date is long forgotten, cosmetics were part of the daily routine of various tribes and cultures around the world. Some used them to increase their beauty, while others applied them as symbolic protection from various threats.

FOR TRADITIONAL KOREAN SOCIETY, COSMETICS HAVE ALWAYS HAD A DEEPER MEANING. Koreans traditionally believed that physical appearance reflected the interior person. For this reason, Korean men and women have always sought to present themselves at their best and have thus created a unique culture. Remember this anecdote when someone tells you that your interest in cosmetics is skin deep!

17

The history of make-up and cosmetics in Korea began during the Three Kings era, which lasted more than seven hundred years (57BCE–668CE). Cosmetic products certainly existed at this time, and were stored in magnificent containers made principally from clay. The high point for cosmetics was reached during the Goryeo dynasty (918–1392), when people began to take even greater interest in personal care and physical appearance. Moreover, Korea was opening up to foreign trade, which allowed new ingredients and techniques to be introduced to the country.

After the fall of Goryeo, the Joseon dynasty was established. During this period (1392–1897), and in accordance with the values of Confucianism, where balance and harmony were key, the use of strident make-up was restricted. Abundance and extremes were disdained in favour of more natural make-up. However, no such restrictions applied to the containers for cosmetics and accessories: beautifully crafted little blue and white porcelain boxes were made for storing make-up, mirrors, combs and other personal grooming items.

**DID YOU KNOW? Korea's name is derived from the Goryeo/Koryŏ dynasty.**

Let's make a small detour to the world of today. What do you consider when you're putting on make-up? You probably have a model or a vlogger you base your routine on, right? Well, it was just the same during the Joseon dynasty. Elite ladies would adapt trends established by *gisaeng*, women artists who dedicated themselves to entertaining the kings.

Nonetheless, cosmetics didn't really come into fashion for a wider audience until the 19th century, when they began to be distributed and purchased on a large scale. New styles and products were developed, many of them inspired by Western culture.

CAN YOU GUESS THE FIRST MASS-PRODUCED COSMETIC TO BE USED IN KOREA? No, it wasn't a cream or face mask, but rather *Bakgabun* (Park's powder), a sort of translucent face powder created in 1915 that was a bestseller for years. There's no point in looking for it now because it's been withdrawn from the market due to its high lead content. However, alternatives with better ingredients soon came onto the market. You wouldn't expect any less from the Koreans, would you?

From the 1920s right through to the 1950s there wasn't much innovation in Korean cosmetics because Japanese products dominated the market. Actually, it's complicated to speak about this period as Japanese occupation and the Second World War dominated Korea. One positive development during that time was the founding of AmorePacific, a beauty conglomerate that has since become one of the best known cosmetic firms in the world.

SO HOW DID KOREAN COSMETICS BECOME AN INTERNATIONAL PHENOMENON? The hype about K-beauty has arrived in the West only very recently, in the last decade or so, and it all began with BB cream. Can you remember life without this miraculous product?

In fact, BB cream is a German invention, but it became extremely popular in Korea, and various cosmetic brands perfected the formula for the national market. The Korean formulation began to be sold in the United States in 2011, and arrived in Spain a few months later. This product was the first wave of the tsunami of

Korean cosmetics in the Western world. Suddenly women had access to the 'affordable luxury' of single-use face masks, containers with fun Asian aesthetics and innovative ingredients such as snail slime extract and bee venom (more of this on page 116). How could anyone resist?

In the years following the BB cream revolution, online shops began a flourishing trade in selected K-beauty products. We opened the doors of our first MiiN shop in 2014, and although we loved the hand cream in apple-shaped containers, the colourful masks and the facial mists in the shape of bunny rabbits, we were truly convinced by the results of these products. Behind the adorable packaging, there is a wealth of effective and original natural ingredients – everything from bamboo carbon powder and donkey milk to bird's nest and algae – almost any ingredient you could imagine! Obviously, Korean cosmetics are here to stay. Anyone who tries the ten-step Korean skincare routine will immediately fall in love with it. Learning to respect, love and care for your skin is the essence of K-beauty!

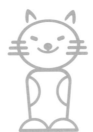

# HOW THE K-BEAUTY PHENOMENON BEGAN

KOREAN COSMETICS ARE MUCH MORE THAN A COMMERCIAL PHENOMENON; THEY'RE A LIFESTYLE. The Korean skincare routine isn't just ten steps you have to follow – it's a ritual, an art. Actually, as well as being great and appealing products, Korean cosmetics have reached the top because they are based on a philosophy that can be applied to many aspects of life.

21

For Koreans, beauty is very important and starts from inside. Avoiding skin imperfections is more important than covering them up with make-up. Consequently, facial treatments are the basis for the routine and the most important step.

KOREAN CULTURE, TRADITIONS AND LIFESTYLE REFLECT THE IMPORTANCE GIVEN TO BEAUTY. Everything is cared for carefully, from public spaces to interpersonal relationships, and skin is treated with the same respect.

**There is an entire philosophy at the heart of the Korean beauty routine which can be applied to many aspects of life.**

However, beyond cultural customs and a taste for beauty, there are other factors that have turned K-beauty into an international phenomenon. We can't forget the popularity and success of K-pop (music) and K-drama (soap operas). As Korean singers and actors are becoming better known in the Western world through social media, the general public is becoming more and more interested in the products they use and the clothing brands they favour.

Due to the internet and social media, we are learning more rapidly about the fashions of other countries. Trends are created and achieve success almost instantaneously. In South Korea, the influence of K-pop groups and the actors in TV programmes for young people is such that they often front advertising campaigns for the major cosmetic brands. It's easy to find their faces on the packaging, in television advertising and related merchandising. These individuals serve as reference points, and their immaculate skin is desired by teenagers and adults alike.

Another contributing factor in the popularity of K-beauty lies in the technical advances made by the Korean cosmetic industry. It has been able to develop totally innovative products that don't exist in other markets, such as splash masks, hydrogel patches for eyes and lips, fluid make-up cushions and sheet masks. All have a part to play in our daily beauty routine, and they have attracted worldwide attention, with Western brands now trying to produce their own formulations for the European and American markets. Apart from their effectiveness, the products are high in quality and low in price, which has no doubt contributed to them spreading across the globe like wildfire.

ONE OF THE PRINCIPAL OBJECTIVES OF KOREAN BRANDS IS TO APPEAL TO YOUNG CLIENTS. In general, Korean women begin to look after their skin from a young age, something they learn from their mothers. Indeed, some brands are especially designed for young (even very young) people. Etude House, for example, markets to teenagers around the age of 15. This, along with the influence of celebrities on screen and in advertising, means that cosmetic treatments are used at a younger and younger age. In fact, several brands have had to lower their target consumer age from 40 to 20.

**Innovations in Korean cosmetics have captured the world's attention.**

# 02

---

# THE IMPORTANCE
# OF CARING FOR
# YOUR SKIN
## 스킨케어의중요성

---

CARING FOR YOUR SKIN IS NOT JUST A QUESTION OF IMAGE. Skin is the protective barrier that acts like a shield to protect the body from any exterior attack or threat. Our ultimate objective in applying a treatment is therefore to care for the skin and keep it healthy, not just to make it beautiful. With the right beauty routine, the end result will be nothing less than radiant.

SKIN GIVES US SIGNALS AND WE HAVE TO OBSERVE IT IN ORDER TO DO WHAT'S NEEDED. At times, all we have to do is stand in front of a mirror and look carefully at our face. The first thing you will see is an imperfection that requires a specific treatment, such as rosacea, acne or an allergic reaction. In this case, you must start by visiting a dermatologist. Once the issue has been resolved, you can use other cosmetic products to obtain specific benefits.

If you don't have any medical issues, let's return to the mirror. What do you see and what would you like to improve? Would you like your skin to be clearer? Are you worried about your first wrinkles? Do you perceive dullness? Would you like your skin to be dewier? Cosmetics must never be used without knowing your skin type, so this is the first step to finding a routine that is right for your needs. You should continue observing your skin on a regular basis because it varies in different circumstances: winter to summer, and during stressful and relaxing times. Remember, everyone's skin is different, so don't just use the same products as someone else. Examine your skin every day when you perform your beauty routine, and observe what it needs. It will thank you.

HOW DO I KNOW WHAT KIND OF SKIN I HAVE? I've lost track of how many times I have been asked this question! It's true that sometimes it's difficult to know your skin type, especially if you consider the different issues that can arise from person to person. Let's begin with some basic concepts, and by the end of this chapter you will be an expert in this subject.

Knowing your skin is the first step to finding a routine that's right for you.

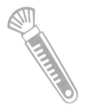

# SKIN TYPES

Skin can be classified into three types: oily, dry and combination. We could add 'normal' skin to this list, but PRACTICALLY NO ONE'S SKIN IS NORMAL. Around 90 per cent of those who believe their skin is normal actually have combination skin. Let's look at each type in turn.

OILY SKIN ARISES FROM THE OVER-PRODUCTION OF SEBUM. Sebum is the oil generated by the sebaceous glands. People with this skin type are usually desperate to eliminate shine from their face, especially in the T-zone (forehead, nose and chin). It's a challenge to ensure that make-up remains in place when you have oily skin, as your face can become as slippery as a ski slope! On the other hand, oily skin has the advantage of ageing less. Shine is easier to deal with than wrinkles.

AT THE OTHER END OF THE SPECTRUM IS DRY SKIN, WHICH SUFFERS FROM LACK OF OIL. Levels of oiliness are regulated by the sebaceous glands and, unfortunately, we have to accept that we can't modify our genetics. *C'est la vie!* Dry skin is usually tight and dehydrated, which can be quite uncomfortable, especially after washing. It's also worse in winter, when harsh weather and central heating tend to dry it out even further. Looking on the bright side, people with dry skin don't have to worry about shine. Also, their pores are very tight, which is aesthetically pleasing.

FINALLY, COMBINATION SKIN HAS THE CHARACTERISTICS OF BOTH OILY AND DRY SKIN. The T-zone can be oily, while the cheeks tend to be drier. The key is to find the right products (or combination of products) for this skin type, which can be quite a challenge. Don't worry, though – as this is the most common skin type and so there are many solutions available.

Hopefully, you will now have a clearer idea of what skin type you're dealing with. But what if you're still a little confused because your skin type isn't described here? The answer is that you probably have a particular issue or skin condition. Let's look at those now.

# THE MOST COMMON SKIN PROBLEMS

01

ACNE

This condition, which is caused by inflamed or infected sebaceous glands, isn't just a problem for those with oily skin. People with dry skin can also have acne. Specific Korean treatments are ideal for improving and preventing this condition because they contain very effective natural ingredients (see Chapter 5, page 113) that help prevent imperfections, reduce outbreaks and repair acne scars. It's very important not to forget hydration during the facial routine. Even though it can be tempting to let the skin dry out a little in order to dry out your pimples, remember that when the skin is dry, the sebaceous glands generate even more oil.

## 02

### SENSITIVITY

This is a very common issue because every skin type can suffer from it. Sensitivity, which can manifest as redness and rashes, is most often caused by an adverse reaction to cosmetic products, or by external factors such as temperature and pollution. Sensitive skin just needs a little extra attention, and we have to test what works and what doesn't. If you want to try new products, you must do so patiently, one by one, in order to avoid unexpected results.

## 03

### HYPERPIGMENTATION

This problem appears when the skin produces excessive melanin, the pigment that gives our skin its colour. The result is dark patches or spots. The best prevention is a good sun cream, such as the Korean products created specifically to treat this condition.

## 04

### AGEING

We all get older – that's life! The ageing process actually begins in your twenties, when the production of collagen decreases. This means that the skin begins to lose hydration and elasticity, though the effects aren't perceived until much later. If you have mature skin, you must continue with specific treatments for your skin type and add some anti-ageing products to your skincare routine to stimulate the production of collagen. (While you're about it, why not include some products with a lifting effect?) Don't forget that the best prevention against wrinkles is to always apply sun cream with a high sun protection factor (SPF).

# HOW TO DISCOVER
# YOUR SKIN TYPE

We hope that you are beginning to understand the differences between the various skin types, but here is a way of discovering your skin type if you still aren't sure:

01
Wash your face as you would normally (if you use the double-cleansing technique as described on pages 38–45, then that's even better).

02
Once you've finished, don't apply any product.

03
Wait approximately one hour, then look at yourself in the mirror. What do you see? If your complexion is shiny and appears greasy, you probably have oily skin. If it's greasy only in the T-zone, you have combination skin. If the skin feels right and there's no greasiness, you have dry skin. *Voilà!*

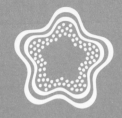

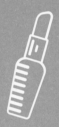

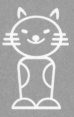

# 03

---

## KOREAN BEAUTY PRODUCTS
한국의 미용 제품

---

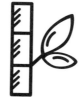

Before we enter the fabulous world of Korean cosmetics and learn what each of them can do for your skin, let's review the various types of products that can be found on the market. You will have heard about many of these items, and you will certainly have used some of them, but when used in combination, it's vital to know their individual importance within the beauty routine. Once you are armed with this information, you will know how to combine them to do the very best for your skin.

# CLEANSING OIL
## 오일 클렌징

**CLEANSING, THE FIRST STEP IN THE KOREAN SKINCARE ROUTINE, IS FUNDAMENTAL. UNFORTUNATELY, MANY PEOPLE SKIP IT.**

Using a cleansing oil is also the first step in the famous Korean double-cleansing technique, going together like socks and shoes or shampoo and conditioner. This step prepares the skin for the Korean beauty ritual that we enjoy so much, so let us explain how this product will change your life.

### DESCRIPTION

The name says it all: cleansing oil is a cleanser formulated with ingredients based on oil. This doesn't mean that it's like washing your face with olive oil. Actually, the oils used are specially formulated for facial skin so that they emulsify better and are easier to remove. Some of the most common ingredients used in these cleansers are jojoba seed, flax, onagri, argan, macadamia nut, coconut and sunflower seed oil, but there are many others. Cleansing oils nourish the skin, and their texture is very pleasant: as they are vegetable oils, they slide onto the skin like silk.

Cleansing oil has a 'magnetic effect', lifting out sebum, oily make-up and sun cream that have accumulated in the pores, something that no water-based cleanser can do, however good it may be. Thus, if your skin is too oily, you will be able to remove all the excess sebum and dirt. The result? Clean, soft and silky skin. Those who suffer from acne have fallen in love with this step precisely because it allows them to prevent and control outbreaks.

—
METHOD OF USE
—

We know what you're thinking: 'Why should I put oil on my face if I'm trying to decrease oiliness?' It may come as a surprise, but oil-based cleansers are very effective on oily and combination skin.

These cleansers are available in a wide range of formulations, so you can easily find something that suits your needs. The most popular ones come in a small canister with a manual pump, and you need use only a couple of drops as it is very concentrated.

Alternatively, you may also have seen cleansing balms, which come in small jars with a spatula for application. Balms have a thicker appearance, but they melt in contact with the skin, so are very easy to use and also feel quite luxurious. Alternatively, if you are always in a hurry, you can use a cleansing bar – very practical for carrying in your gym bag or using on your travels. Just twist off about a centimetre of product and apply it to your face.

How to apply a cleansing oil:

01 Apply a few drops of oil onto dry skin, or a pea-sized amount of balm onto wet skin, and massage with circular movements so that the magnetic effect works all over your face. Enjoy this moment of relaxing massage.

02 Splash the face with tepid water, taking care to remove the cleanser thoroughly, as some brands require more time than others (it also depends on the quantity of sebum and dirt to be removed).

03 Dry with a clean towel.

—
MYTH-BUSTING
—

Cleansing oils are great for any skin type: they hydrate mature and dry skin, they reduce the sebum of oily skin, and their gentle formulations usually work well with sensitive skin. This is good news because they are the only way to ensure you have removed all your make-up before proceeding to the double-cleansing process.

A certain amount of confusion surrounds the best time to use a cleansing oil. Many people think it should be used only at night to remove make-up and sun cream. Of course, it's really important to clean your face well at the end of the day, but cleansing it in the morning too will help to keep your skin radiant. That's because your skin continues to generate sebum while you sleep, and your face will accumulate different particles (such as oil) from contact with the pillow. Consequently, deep-cleansing your skin in the morning as the first step of your facial routine is the ideal way to begin the day. Have we convinced you yet?

## WHAT WE LIKE ABOUT CLEANSING OILS

- ♥ THEY ARE A PLEASURE TO USE.
- ♥ THEY ARE PERFECT FOR ALL SKIN TYPES, ESPECIALLY OILY SKIN.
- ♥ THEY LEAVE THE SKIN SOFT AND READY FOR THE REST OF YOUR BEAUTY ROUTINE.
- ♥ YOU WILL SEE INSTANT RESULTS.

## OUR FAVOURITES

- ♥ *GENTLE BLACK DEEP CLEANSING OIL* BY KLAIRS.
- ♥ *ORANGE CLEANSING SHERBET* BY AROMATICA.
- ♥ *ULTRA WATERY EOSEONGCHO CLEANSER* BY A. BY BOM.

## SUMMARY

USING A CLEANSING OIL IS THE FIRST STEP IN THE KOREAN SKINCARE ROUTINE. IT ELIMINATES IMPURITIES, SUCH AS SEBUM AND MAKE-UP, LEAVING THE SKIN AS CLEAR AS A FRESH, WHITE SHEET.

## TIP

We love it when packaging is decorated with pandas, but dark circles around our eyes don't look as good as on these cute animals. In order to remove eye make-up completely, moisten a cotton wool pad with cleansing oil and smooth it over the eyelashes to dissolve even the most stubborn mascara and eyeliner.

41

# WATER-BASED CLEANSER
## 클렌징폼

**NOW THAT THE CLEANSING OIL HAS GIVEN YOU PURER AND CLEARER SKIN, THE NEXT STEP IS TO USE A WATER-BASED CLEANSER.**

Like the froth on a good cappuccino is essential to the coffee, the creamy foam of a water-based cleanser is the essential second step of the double-cleansing routine. As with cleansing oil, a water-based cleanser removes oil, make-up and sun cream, but its main objective is to eliminate all water-based impurities, such as sweat or different types of contaminating particles. You have probably been doing this step for most of your life, but you will be surprised how combining it with the previous step (cleansing oil, see pages 38–41) increases its effectiveness. Your face will feel truly clean and ready for the remaining steps of the skincare routine.

## DESCRIPTION

—

Yes, you've guessed it – this is a cleanser made principally from water. There are water-based cleansers for every skin type, as well as some for specific skin issues, such as acne outbreaks, dilated pores, dryness and hyperpigmentation. Chapter 5 (see page 113) discusses the formulations in more detail and suggests the best ingredients for every situation.

Cleansing foams have a very liquid consistency, but when you press the manual pump, they magically become a cushion of foam in your hand. We love the lightness of these cleansing foams and how the bubbles spread so easily over the face when they come into contact with the skin.

Gel cleansers are also available, and (as the name suggests) have a thicker, more gelatinous texture. Apply to wet skin and the slippery gel will transform into a very pleasant foam.

If you prefer basic products or a vintage approach, why not try a bar of soap? That's right – a block of water-based cleanser (we promise you it's nothing like your grandmother's soap used to be). Korean facial soaps are carefully created by experts in the cosmetic sector and contain all the ingredients necessary to deeply replenish your skin. It you're on a limited budget, you may well prefer these bars of soap because they last for a very long time.

—

## METHOD OF USE

—

You might not think that there's much to learn about using one of these cleansers, but how do you know if you've been doing it right all these years?

How to apply a water-based cleanser:

01 Wet the face with tepid water. The water temperature is important because if it's too cold, it will be more difficult to clean the pores deeply. On the other hand, if it's too hot, you could damage the skin's natural hydration barrier.

02 Apply a little of the product to your fingers and massage over the face, making upwards circular movements to create a foam.

03 Remove by splashing gently with tepid water.

04 Dry with a clean towel and your skin will look like new!

—
MYTH-BUSTING
—

'It's enough to wash your face with a single type of cleanser.' We've already smashed this very common myth, haven't we? One more time: it's best to begin with a cleansing oil and then wash the face with a water-based cleanser.

We've spoken about the importance of water temperature, but if we were to visit your bathroom, where would we find your cleanser? If it's in your shower, you're doing it wrong! Washing your face in the shower may be practical, but the water is too hot and the pressure is too strong, so use your sink instead.

Another common error is that some people avoid water-based cleansers at all costs because they fear they will dry out their skin. Poor-quality cleansers might do this, but it won't happen with Korean cosmetics! Their excellent formulations with natural ingredients mean that these products will nurture and clean your skin, leaving it healthy and hydrated, which is the whole point of the double-cleansing routine. If you have dry skin, try using a hydrating cleanser – there are lots of options available.

## WHAT WE LIKE ABOUT WATER-BASED CLEANSERS

♥ THE FOAM MADE BY THESE CLEANSERS IS LIKE A BUBBLE BATH FOR THE FACE. INCLUDING THEM IN YOUR ROUTINE WILL BECOME THE BEST PART OF YOUR DAY!

♥ JUST LIKE A PROFESSIONAL TREATMENT, WATER-BASED CLEANSERS WILL REMOVE ALL IMPURITIES FROM YOUR FACE, LEAVING THE SKIN EXTRA CLEAN.

♥ THERE ARE A WIDE VARIETY OF CLEANSERS AVAILABLE, SO YOU CAN FIND A PERFECT OPTION FOR EVERY ISSUE OR SKIN TYPE.

## OUR FAVOURITES

♥ *WHITE IN MILK WHIPPING FOAM* BY G9SKIN.

♥ *RICH MOIST FOAMING CLEANSER* BY KLAIRS.

♥ *HONEST CLEANSING FOAM* BY BENTON.

## SUMMARY

WATER-BASED CLEANSERS ELIMINATE IMPURITIES, MAKE-UP, PERSPIRATION AND CONTAMINATING PARTICLES. THEY WILL MAKE YOUR SKIN LOOK RADIANT!

## TIP

For an even deeper clean, let the foam sink in for a minute before washing it off. This way, the bubbles will have time to act inside your pores.

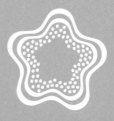

# EXFOLIANT
## 스크럽

**EXFOLIATION – THE REMOVAL
OF DEAD SKIN CELLS – IS A
VITAL PART OF THE KOREAN
SKINCARE ROUTINE.**

Here's a secret: if you feel a little intimidated by all of the steps of the Korean skincare routine (see Chapter 4, pages 107–108), don't worry. You don't have to do all of these steps every day. Exfoliation is one of those steps that is only done occasionally.

The frequency of exfoliation depends on your skin type and the product you use. Exfoliating your face is like cleaning a diamond. There are many different methods of exfoliation. All of them will leave your skin shining and with a perfect texture.

### DESCRIPTION

An exfoliant is a product that removes dead skin cells from the skin and unifies its texture. As scientists tell us, the skin is constantly renewing itself: skin cells are produced in the inner layers of the epidermis and rise to the surface of the skin, the corneal layer. Over time, these cells die and fall off, but exfoliation accelerates the process of elimination, which prevents the skin looking dull.

There are two types of exfoliation, mechanical and chemical, both of which are described below:

MECHANICAL EXFOLIATION is the more common process. It involves using a product with small particles to rub off dead cells. The result is fresh and radiant skin.

CHEMICAL EXFOLIATION uses an acid-based liquid to weaken the lipids that bond the top layers of skin together, thus eliminating dead skin cells. Korean chemical exfoliants tend to use either alpha-hydroxyl acid (AHA) or beta-hydroxyl acid (BHA). The word 'acid' might sound alarming, but the products are quite safe as long as you follow the directions for use. You've probably already used one without even knowing it!

Some examples of AHA are lactic acid, glycolic acid (made from sugar cane) and vegetable enzymes from fruit extracts, such as apple, papaya and pineapple. AHA works the surface more than BHA and is a fantastic option to treat wrinkles and sun-damaged skin. If you have oily skin or suffer sporadic outbreaks of acne, BHA will be your best friend. Anyone who suffered from acne as a teenager knows what makes BHA so popular: salicylic acid. It penetrates the pores to dissolve sebum and dirt, leaving the skin radiant and the pores reduced in size. The results will surprise you!

A word of warning: you must be careful with chemical exfoliants and avoid abusing acids or using them if it isn't necessary. They must not be combined with other aggressive ingredients or those with high proportions of other acids, as this can damage or dry the skin. AHA and BHA can be used together without any problem, as long as you don't overdo it. Start by trying them a couple of nights a week and observe how your skin reacts. If you use them in the morning, do apply a sun cream afterwards because the acids reduce the skin's natural protection from the sun.

## METHOD OF USE

The two types of exfoliant require different methods of application, as explained below.

How to apply a mechanical exfoliant:

01 After double-cleansing, massage a little of the exfoliant onto wet facial skin, avoiding the eyes.
02 Rinse off with tepid water.

How to apply a chemical exfoliant:

01 After double-cleansing, use a cotton wool pad to apply the exfoliant to the face, avoiding the eye area.
02 Wait for the product to dry and proceed with the remaining steps of the facial routine.

## MYTH-BUSTING

Not all mechanical exfoliants are the same, so it's important to check the ingredients before making a purchase. Avoid those containing particles of seeds or fruit husks, as they are too coarse for delicate facial skin and can scratch the outer layer. For the same reason, never use body exfoliants on the face.

If you know how to use them, exfoliants are not aggressive. A mechanical exfoliant can be used once a week on normal or dry skin, or up to twice a week on oily or combination skin.

48

If you suffer from acne, do not use a mechanical exfoliant after an outbreak as it will only irritate the skin further. Alternating different types of exfoliant will radically improve your appearance.

## WHAT WE LIKE ABOUT EXFOLIANTS

♥ THERE IS NOTHING LIKE THE SENSORY EXPERIENCE OF A MECHANICAL EXFOLIANT!

♥ CHEMICAL EXFOLIANTS ARE EASY TO USE AND ACHIEVE MIRACLES WITH BLACKHEADS AND PIMPLES, AS WELL AS GIVING NEW LIFE TO TIRED SKIN.

## OUR FAVOURITES

♥ *GENTLE BLACK SUGAR FACIAL POLISH* BY KLAIRS.

♥ *AHA PEELING LIQUID (HONEY & PROPOLIS)* BY COMMLEAF.

♥ *PATTING SPLASH MASK (GREEN TEA)* BY BLITHE.

## SUMMARY

EXFOLIATION WILL ALLOW YOU TO GET RID OF DEAD SKIN CELLS SO THAT THE PRODUCTS YOU APPLY IN THE REMAINING STEPS OF THE BEAUTY ROUTINE ARE ABSORBED MORE EASILY. IT ALSO HELPS TO MAINTAIN RADIANT AND CLEAR SKIN.

# CLEANSING MASK
클렌징 팩

**TODAY'S KOREAN CLEANSING MASKS ARE NOTHING LIKE THOSE OF YESTERYEAR.**

Let's confront some stereotypes! When you think about a skincare routine, do you think of a girl in a bathrobe, with her hair tied back and a green or white product all over her face? If this is the image you have in your mind, you already know what a wash-off cleansing mask is. Today's Korean masks have nothing to do with those old-fashioned products. We'll bring you up to date!

### DESCRIPTION

Usually made from some type of clay, cleansing masks penetrate the pores to remove impurities and excess sebum. Their objective is to cleanse pores deeply and make them less visible. They have the texture of a paste and usually come in tubes or jars. As they dry out, they solidify and absorb impurities from the face (including blackheads and spots). When you remove the mask with water, everything you don't want on your face is washed away.

Bubble masks are a new type of product – a foam applied to the face so that its oxygen bubbles enter the pores, before being rinsed off. They are much lighter than clay masks and great fun! However, whatever type of cleansing mask you choose, always deep-clean the skin before using one (once or twice a week).

## METHOD OF USE

There are many different cleansing masks, so it's very important that you read the product instructions carefully.

How to use a cleansing mask:

01 After double-cleansing, make sure you apply the mask to dry skin, without massaging.

02 Leave it to work for the time recommended by the product, then rinse off with tepid water. Goodbye forever, blackheads!

51

## MYTH-BUSTING

If you have dry skin, you might worry that a cleansing mask of any type will leave your skin as dry as the Sahara Desert. Wrong! As with all Korean beauty products, the ingredients are carefully chosen to give the best results. Many clay masks are formulated with nutritive ingredients so that your skin will be full of life after using them. And don't forget that the remaining steps of the beauty routine will be adding whatever you think your skin needs in the way of moisture.

If a mask can reduce pores and remove blackheads, skin should feel tight afterwards, right? Wrong! Tightness indicates that your skin has lost too much hydration. This doesn't happen with Korean masks, which are light years ahead of cheaper products sold in supermarkets.

## WHAT WE LIKE ABOUT CLEANSING MASKS

♥  IN JUST A FEW MINUTES, YOU CAN VISIBLY REDUCE PORE SIZE AND ELIMINATE BLACKHEADS AND IMPURITIES.

♥  USING A MASK FORCES YOU TO RELAX, EVEN IF JUST FOR A FEW MOMENTS.

## OUR FAVOURITES

♥  *PORETOX FRUIT SODA BUBBLE MASK* BY BERRISOM.

♥  *SPARKLING MASK* BY SHANGPREE.

♥  *COLOR CLAY CARBONATED BUBBLE PACK* BY G9SKIN.

## SUMMARY

IF YOU ARE LOOKING FOR A RELAXING WAY TO IMPROVE THE APPEARANCE OF YOUR PORES AND ELIMINATE BLACKHEADS AND IMPERFECTIONS, THERE IS NOTHING BETTER THAN A CLEANSING MASK TO ABSORB OIL AND IMPURITIES AND ELIMINATE THEM FOREVER!

# TONER
# 토너

**THIS STEP IS VERY IMPORTANT,
SO DON'T SKIP IT!**

Light and refreshing like springtime rain or a glass of water with ice and lemon, toner is a fantastic product, and an easy way to make your skin dewier. Hydration is essential for healthy skin, and there is nothing better than moistening with toner to give your skin a good dose of water.

DESCRIPTION

If you've used poor-quality toners in the past, you might think they are only useful to prevent acne or to reduce the size of pores. Even though some do work like this, the principal objective of any Korean toner is to hydrate the skin and balance its pH (acidity). If your skin has a low pH level, you can suffer irritation, redness and acne, while if the pH is too high, it provokes dryness and flaking. We don't want either!

Toners return skin to its ideal state, which corresponds to a pH level of approximately 5. Basically, toner is like yoga in a bottle. Balance is the key!

Another function of toners is that they hydrate the skin enough to help it absorb products even better. Think of skin like a sponge: which absorbs more, a sponge which is dry and half broken, or one which is slightly damp? The second, basically! Using a toner allows the skin to absorb essences, serums, facial oils, lotions and creams. The active ingredients of these treatments will penetrate the pores more efficiently, and this in turn will improve their results.

When choosing a toner, look for sprays that have a manual pump or bottles with an eye dropper because these ensure that the product doesn't spoil and the consistency remains very liquid.

—
METHOD OF USE
—

There are two ways to apply a toner: the traditional method and the alternative Korean method. Choose which option you prefer!

How to apply a toner:

01 After double-cleansing, dry the face.
02 Dampen a cotton wool pad with toner and apply onto the face. Alternatively, for the Korean method, let some drops of toner fall into the palm of the hand, and use light touches to dab it over the face, gently massaging it in until absorbed.

Believe it or not, rubbing the face with a cotton pad will lightly exfoliate it, so sensitive skin can become slightly irritated. In this case, opt for using the Korean technique. What makes this Korean?

The gentle touch, of course! Applying products with soft touches on the skin is a delicate method that avoids damaging the skin and delays the appearance of wrinkles.

Light touches must also be used with the *7 Skin Method* (see page 154). The Korean language uses the same word for 'skin' and 'toner', so the 7 *Skin Method* simply consists in applying toner seven times. When your skin needs intensive hydration (either because the air conditioning in the office has dried it out or because you want to look your best at a special event), it's time for toner! You can use the same toner seven times or combine different types, always starting with the lightest consistency and ending with the heaviest. Simply apply one layer, using some light touches with the fingers for it to absorb, then repeat until you have done it seven times. The results will surprise you!

—

MYTH-BUSTING

—

A good toner doesn't have to sting or provoke tightness – on the contrary! Korean toners hydrate the skin after double-cleansing so that it is dewy and ready to absorb the active ingredients of the products that follow. Moreover, if you want to generate less residue, opt for the Korean method of application (see step 2, page 55) – be sure to apply it to the face with light touches.

## WHAT WE LIKE ABOUT TONERS

♥ THEIR LIGHT AND LIQUID TEXTURE IS VERY REFRESHING. IF YOUR SKIN COULD SIGH WITH PLEASURE, IT WOULD!

♥ THEY ABSORB VERY RAPIDLY AND USING LIGHT TOUCHES TO APPLY THEM FEELS LIKE A MASSAGE.

## OUR FAVOURITES

♥ *ALOE BHA SKIN TONER* BY BENTON.

♥ *SUPPLE PREPARATION FACIAL TONER* BY KLAIRS.

♥ *ULTRA BOTANIC SKIN WATER* BY A. BY BOM.

## SUMMARY

DON'T BE MISLED BY THE LIGHT TEXTURE OF TONERS; THEY ARE REALLY EFFECTIVE IN BALANCING THE pH LEVELS OF YOUR SKIN. WHEN YOU HYDRATE WITH A TONER, YOU'RE ALSO PREPARING YOUR SKIN TO GET MAXIMUM ABSORPTION OF THE PRODUCTS APPLIED AFTERWARDS. USE TONER AND YOUR SKIN WILL THANK YOU!

## TIP

If you're looking for some extra hydration and don't have a single-use face mask to hand, make your own by placing toner on one or two cotton wool pads and leave them on your face for five to ten minutes.

# FACIAL MIST
## 미스트

**IF YOU STILL HAVEN'T UNDERSTOOD THAT HYDRATION IS KEY IN THE KOREAN BEAUTY ROUTINE, THIS STEP WILL LEAVE YOU WITH NO FURTHER DOUBTS.**

Even if you follow all the Korean skincare routine steps and begin each morning with a radiant face, it's inevitable that your skin will lose hydration during the day. Thank goodness for facial mist, a very simple treatment that leaves skin hydrated, elastic and full of life!

### DESCRIPTION

Facial mist is used when you need a touch of hydration. If you want to purchase one with some other product from the routine, the most similar is toner, though some mists have higher concentrations of active ingredients. You can also use mists alongside an essence or a serum.

Without doubt, misting is the easiest step of the entire Korean beauty routine, as you only have to spray a little of the product on the face and you're ready! Are you going to the gym in the morning? Refresh your skin with a facial mist after a workout. Have you spent all day in the office with air conditioning or heating on full blast? A little facial mist will keep your skin hydrated. Have you agreed to a last-minute date and you want a special shine? You already know what you have to do...

How to apply a facial mist:

01 After applying toner, spray the mist on your face. Wait ten seconds, then use light touches of your fingers to pat it into the skin until absorbed into the face.

02 You can also use facial mist to set make-up. Just apply it when you're done!

03 Apply mist whenever the skin needs a dose of hydration.

MYTH-BUSTING

'A facial mist is nothing more than water in a bottle, it's not worth buying.' Even though it's true that some of the first facial mists were advertised as mineral waters, they have evolved a great deal since then. Look at the list of ingredients on the bottle and choose a facial mist with active ingredients.

'My skin is too oily to use a mist,' or 'My skin is so dry that I need a stronger product.' First of all, even if you have oily skin, it's also likely to be dehydrated. Excessive production of sebum is the reaction of oily skin to a lack of hydration, so facial mist is a very good option (there are even matte mists that can reduce shine). If your skin is very dry, you need an ultra-hydrating facial mist. Any mist with hyaluronic acid will be perfect for you.

## WHAT WE LIKE ABOUT FACIAL MISTS

- THEY ARE EASY TO CARRY AROUND, SO YOU CAN USE THEM WHEREVER YOU GO AND WHENEVER YOU WISH.
- THEY ARE THE PERFECT PRODUCT TO REFRESH YOUR SKIN WHEN IT NEEDS HYDRATION.
- THE SENSATION OF MIST ON THE SKIN FEELS FANTASTIC!

## OUR FAVOURITES

- *ROSE BLOOMING MIST* BY COMMLEAF.
- *BEAUTY WATER* BY SON & PARK (THIS COMES IN AN ORDINARY BOTTLE, SO WE RECOMMEND THAT YOU DECANT SOME INTO A SMALL SPRAY BOTTLE AND ALWAYS CARRY IT WITH YOU).
- *PERFECT DAILY MIST* BY URANG.

## SUMMARY

CARRYING A FACIAL MIST IN YOUR BAG SHOWS THAT THE KOREAN BEAUTY RITUAL IS PART OF YOUR LIFESTYLE. USE IT TO ADD SOME HYDRATION TO YOUR ROUTINE AFTER YOU APPLY TONER, AND REMEMBER THAT YOU CAN REPEAT IT AT ANY TIME DURING THE DAY.

# ESSENCE
에센스

**THERE IS SOMETHING MAGICAL
AND MYSTERIOUS ABOUT THIS
BEAUTY PRODUCT.**

The word 'essence' has almost spiritual connotations, suggesting the intrinsic nature of something, and conveying a sense of magic and mystery. Let's discover what has made half the world fall in love with this product.

DESCRIPTION

As you have learned, the objective of toners is to hydrate the skin and balance its pH, so think of an essence as a high-powered version of that treatment, containing such a concentration of the active ingredients that the results are greatly multiplied. Do you need more hydration? Want to reduce wrinkles? You're in luck, because there's an essence for everything! Essences don't have cleansing properties, but if you take a quick look at their composition, you will see how effective they can be.

This step is simple, as essence is applied just like a toner. It can be patted onto the skin using light touches, or – even easier – can be decanted into a spray bottle and applied over the face.

There are three ways to apply an essence:

01 After applying a toner and waiting for it to absorb, apply the essence following the same method of application.
02 Alternatively, pour a little essence onto a cotton wool pad or directly in the palm of your hand and apply it with soft touches to the skin.
03 Spray the essence over the face and dab it in with your fingers until completely absorbed.

63

The consistency will vary greatly from one essence to another: some are very liquid, while others are more like gels. Don't worry too much about consistency, as the ingredients it contains are more important.

There is a great deal of confusion about essences in the Western world due to lack of information. Despite their consistency, they are nothing like a cleanser. They are applied as one of the intermediary steps of the beauty routine (after toner and before serum) and should be used before applying make-up so that the active ingredients can penetrate the pores. We like to say that an essence is like a fruit nectar – a mixture of vitamins and nutrition for your skin!

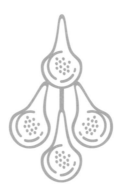

## WHAT WE LIKE ABOUT ESSENCES

- THEIR VERY HIGH CONCENTRATION OF ACTIVE INGREDIENTS PROVIDES VISIBLE RESULTS.
- THEY ADD A LAYER OF HYDRATION TO FACIAL SKIN – VERY IMPORTANT, AS WE MUST PROTECT OUR HYDRATION BARRIER AS MUCH AS POSSIBLE!

## OUR FAVOURITES

- *VITAL TREATMENT 9 ESSENTIALS SEEDS* BY BLITHE.
- *SNAIL BEE HIGH CONTENT ESSENCE* BY BENTON.
- *BIRCH JUICE HYDRO ESSENCE SKIN* BY E NATURE.

## SUMMARY

ESSENCES HAVE BECOME AN ESSENTIAL PRODUCT IN KOREA AS THEY ARE THE KEY TO ACHIEVING (AND MAINTAINING) A SHINE. IT'S A VERY EASY STEP TO ADD TO YOUR FACIAL ROUTINE AND WILL GIVE YOU 'PRO' STATUS WITH COSMETICS!

# SERUM
세럼

**A MIRACULOUS LIQUID
IN A SMALL BOTTLE.**

We don't know what you think, but we associate this product with luxury, perhaps because a single drop of serum has such a concentration of ingredients that it seems like liquid gold. Perhaps you have also heard about ampoules, which are tiny containers of even more concentrated forms of serum. Whatever format you prefer, the serum is used in exactly the same way.

DESCRIPTION

If you want to address a particular issue – perhaps how to highlight your face, reduce wrinkles or eliminate imperfections – serum is the product for you. Its small molecules penetrate easily into the pores, allowing active ingredients to reach deep into the skin. Serums are light because they are water-based. This means they are absorbed in a matter of seconds and leave a very fresh sensation.

The key to successful application lies in using the correct quantity and applying it with care. There are different ways to apply a serum, but they are all equally effective.

How to apply a serum:

01 After double-cleansing, then applying toner and essence, place some drops of serum in the hand.

02 Apply to the cheeks, chin and forehead and massage gently, using soft touches with your fingers so that the skin absorbs the serum.

An alternative method consists of mixing some drops of serum with your day cream and then applying it to the face. This technique works well if you are trying a new serum, especially one that has an active ingredient, such as vitamin A, that can sometimes irritate sensitive skin. If your skin reacts well to the mixture, you can place the serum directly on your face the next time you use it.

MYTH-BUSTING

'All serums are expensive and don't last.' How many times have we heard this? If you use the serum correctly, every small bottle should last! The formula of these products is so concentrated that a few drops are more than sufficient to achieve the results you want. Four drops is enough, so use an eye dropper to release just the required amount. With regard to price, a serum is usually a little more expensive than a cleanser or toner because its ingredients are stronger and therefore last longer. But you're worth it, right?

## WHAT WE LIKE ABOUT SERUMS

- YOU CAN DO SO MUCH WITH SO LITTLE, EVEN WITH JUST A FEW DROPS, BECAUSE OF ITS CONCENTRATION.
- SERUM IS SMALL BUT IT PACKS A MIGHTY PUNCH!
- IT SLIDES OVER THE FACE IN A VERY PLEASING WAY.

## OUR FAVOURITES

- *FRESHLY JUICED VITAMIN DROP* BY KLAIRS.
- *ROSE ABSOLUTE FIRST SERUM* BY AROMATICA.
- *VITAMIN OIL SERUM* BY URANG.

## SUMMARY

SMALL YET POWERFUL IS THE BEST WAY TO DESCRIBE SERUMS. WATER-BASED AND FILLED WITH ACTIVE INGREDIENTS, THEY ARE PERFECT FOR TREATING SPECIFIC ISSUES. YOU WILL ALSO FEEL MARVELLOUS FOR SPOILING YOUR SKIN LIKE THIS.

# SINGLE-USE FACE MASK
팩

**THE STAR OF THE KOREAN SKINCARE ROUTINE.**

If we had to choose a product to define Korean cosmetics, without doubt it would be the single-use face mask! We're now accustomed to using these masks, but just five years ago it was very rare to hear about them, let alone use them. Nonetheless, Korean women have been using them for the past ten years, at least three times a week (sometimes even daily), and it has become an essential step in their beauty routine. Nowadays, every brand produces its own range of different masks, so there are thousands to choose from. Some tips are needed in order to choose the best one, right?

### DESCRIPTION

There is such a variety of masks available that it is practically impossible to provide a general description. However, they all share the same design feature, as they have been created to completely cover the face and incorporate a thin layer filled with essence. This layer creates a barrier that prevents the product from evaporating, thus allowing the active ingredients to penetrate the skin effectively.

The treatment provided by a mask is very concentrated, so results can be seen rapidly, even though it's not a flashy product. Did you know that a mask contains between 20 and 35 millilitres of essence? In many cases, the ingredients are similar to those found in serums. What a luxury!

Whatever your skin type, age and needs, there will be a perfect mask for you. Their principal function is to hydrate the skin, but increasingly you can find masks that have other functions too: highlighting, anti-ageing, anti-pollution, anti-acne – you name it! For this reason, it is important to check the ingredients carefully before trying them.

Masks can be classified according to their composition, rather than their cosmetic ingredients:

COTTON MASKS are the best known. They are usually white and their texture is similar to cloth. They are soft and porous so that the skin can breathe. Their adherence to the skin is not perfect, so it's difficult to do other things while using them. This means you get 20 minutes of compulsory relaxation!

HYDROGEL MASKS are made with biocompatible polymers and have an extensive system of absorption. The material itself helps to refresh and decongest the skin. Unlike cotton masks, hydrogel masks aren't porous, but they do adhere perfectly to the face, which means you can move around and do other activities while wearing them. (Despite that, our favourite option is still to relax for 20 minutes without doing anything other than spoiling ourselves.) Generally, hydrogel masks are separated into two pieces: one covering the upper part of the face and the other covering the lower part. For ease of application, we recommend beginning with the upper part.

BIO-CELLULOSE MASKS are halfway between hydrogel and cotton in terms of their adherence to the skin. They were designed to improve some aspects of cotton masks and are made from cellulose microbiome, a completely natural fibre offering good absorption. Sheets with the highest bio-cellulose content offer hermetic (airtight) adhesion to the skin, which allows them to transfer cosmetic ingredients very efficiently.

—

METHOD OF USE

—

There are no specific rules, but there are some things that should always be remembered when applying a single-use facial mask. First, it's important to put the mask on clean skin, generally after using toner, essence or serum. This depends on the steps included in your routine.

Second, single-use face masks usually have hydrating properties, so they should never be applied before toner. However, they shouldn't be confused with cleansing masks, which are always applied before any step offering hydration.

Finally, while you can use up to seven single-use face masks a week, the ideal is between three and four, but do always ensure that the ingredients your masks contain are compatible with the rest of the products in your routine. For example, if the mask contains acid, it's better to use it only once a week and look for hydrating masks with hyaluronic acid or collagen for the other days.

How to apply a single-use facial mask:

01 After double-cleansing and using toner, place the mask on the skin.

02 Leave it to work for the amount of time indicated on the product package, then remove it.

03 Massage the product into the skin until fully absorbed.

—
MYTH-BUSTING
—

'If I leave the mask on for longer, I will obtain better results.' Wrong! Increasing the length of time the mask is left in place won't increase the effects. Masks must work for the time indicated, generally 10–30 minutes, no more.

'Masks can be used again.' Actually, this is wrong too. After using them, masks must be thrown away. However, we do have a tip to ensure that you maximise any essence remaining in them: simply use them to hydrate other parts of the body, such as the neck, cleavage, arms or legs.

'I have to wash my face after using them.' Wrong! If you do this, you will cancel out the effect of the mask. Allow the product to be absorbed into the skin before moving on to the remaining steps of the routine.

73

## WHAT WE LIKE ABOUT SINGLE-USE FACE MASKS

♥  THERE ARE SO MANY DIFFERENT ONES TO TRY, AND THEY ARE ECONOMICAL, SO YOU CAN TRY AS MANY AS YOU LIKE.

♥  YOU CAN TAKE THEM ANYWHERE, EVEN ONTO A FLIGHT.

♥  A USED MASK CAN BE APPLIED TO OTHER PARTS OF THE BODY, SUCH AS THE NECK, CLEAVAGE OR ARMS.

## OUR FAVOURITES

♥  *3D VOLUME GUM MASK* BY G9SKIN.

♥  *JUMISO WHOA WHOA SOOTHING MASK* BY HELLO SKIN.

♥  *DON'T WORRY HEALING MASK* BY PACKAGE.

## SUMMARY

SINGLE-USE FACE MASKS ARE LIKE A SECOND SKIN THAT COVERS YOUR FACE AND IMPROVES IT, PRODUCING RADIANT RESULTS IN JUST A FEW MINUTES. THIS IS AN INTENSIVE HYDRATION TREATMENT THAT FITS IN YOUR HANDBAG!

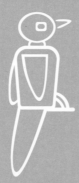

**TIP**
**During the summer,
chill your facial mask
in the refrigerator
for a really
refreshing effect.**

## UNCONVENTIONAL MASKS:

♥ *ULTRA COOL LEAF MASK* BY A. BY BOM
– A TWO-STEP MASK THAT INCLUDES SOME
LEAF-SHAPED PATCHES TO APPLY BELOW
THE MASK IN PLACES SUCH AS THE CHEEKS,
FOREHEAD OR FACIAL CONTOURS.

♥ *WRAPPING ME MOISTURE SAUNA MASK*
BY P:REM – THIS FOIL MASK KEEPS IN THE
HEAT FROM YOUR SKIN AND CREATES A
SAUNA-LIKE EFFECT.

# EYE CREAM
## 아이 크림

**THE SKIN AROUND THE EYES IS UP
TO FIVE TIMES MORE DELICATE
THAN THE SKIN ON THE REST OF
THE BODY, SO IT REQUIRES
GREATER ATTENTION.**

Eye cream deserves special attention. It's not just a marketing strategy; it is formulated specifically for the delicate skin in the eye area, which can be up to five times thinner than skin elsewhere on the body: a mere 0.05–0.1 millimetres – nothing! Nonetheless, it still acts as a protective barrier, so we need to pay it extra attention and care for it with specific products which can even be tolerated by those who have sensitive skin.

We have all made the mistake of thinking that the day cream we use for the face can also be used as an eye cream, but this is wrong because some ingredients can be aggressive and irritate the very delicate eye area. But there's good news! In general, eye creams are formulated with concentrated and very effective ingredients because the skin around the eyes is where the first signs of ageing appear. Note too, that these creams can also be applied to the lips.

Eye cream usually comes in small (15-millilitre) containers, though some brands are more generous and offer 30 millilitres. Both might seem to be tiny amounts, but they are more than sufficient when you consider that a quantity equivalent to a grain of rice is sufficient for treating two eyes.

While eye cream serves principally to treat wrinkles in the eye zone and to brighten dark circles, it can't eliminate them.

Do not confuse dark circles with bags. The latter are formed when oil or liquid accumulates under the eyes, and can be reduced with the use of hydrogel patches. These patches, shaped like half-moons, are made from a gelatinous material that sticks perfectly to the skin and reduces bags and congestion in a matter of minutes. The trick is to keep the patches in the refrigerator and apply them cold, ideally in the morning, so that the results are seen throughout the day.

METHOD OF USE

Eye cream should be applied around each eye as far as the cheekbone and the arch of the eyebrow. The product must not be used close to the tear duct or directly on the eyelid, as the capillaries (tiny blood vessels) in the skin will distribute the active ingredients.

Nor should the cream be rubbed or massaged forcefully. Use just light touches with the fingertips, preferably the ring finger.

How to apply an eye cream:

01 Eye cream can be applied both day and night.

02 It is important to apply eye cream before face cream or hydrating lotion, and not as a final step. The reason: if cream or lotion is applied first, it will form a protective layer that will prevent the skin from correctly absorbing the eye cream.

03 Dab the cream on lightly with the fingertips and avoid rubbing the product to prevent irritation.

—
MYTH-BUSTING
—

Without a doubt, the most common myth is that eye cream is for those with mature skin. It all depends on the formulation, but in fact, it's for everyone because it's important to keep the skin hydrated from an early age and thus prevent premature signs of ageing.

## WHAT WE LIKE ABOUT EYE CREAMS

- THEY USUALLY HAVE A VERY HIGH CONCENTRATION OF ACTIVE INGREDIENTS.
- THE TEXTURE IS VERY PLEASANT.
- THEY CAN ALSO BE APPLIED TO THE LIPS.

## OUR FAVOURITES

- *FERMENTATION EYE CREAM* BY BENTON.
- *ULTRA TIME RETURN EYE SERUM* BY A. BY BOM.
- *ROSE ABSOLUTE EYE CREAM* BY AROMATICA.

## SUMMARY

THE PREVENTION OF WRINKLES STARTS WITH EYE CREAM. IT'S THE BEST COSMETIC PRODUCT TO DEMONSTRATE THAT THERE IS NO CORRELATION BETWEEN QUANTITY AND GOOD RESULTS.

# LOTION
로션

**LOTION IS IMPORTANT FOR EVERYONE, EVEN THOSE WITH OILY OR COMBINATION SKIN.**

We at MiiN must confess that before entering the spellbinding world of Korean cosmetics, lotion didn't interest us at all. Cream seemed more than sufficient, and even if we wanted something lighter, we would look for a slightly less sticky cream. However, Korean cosmetics are sophisticated, and lotion now has a special place in our washbag, whether we have oily or combination skin.

### DESCRIPTION

Lotion, sometimes referred to as emulsion, has the same function as cream: to nourish the skin and maintain an optimum level of hydration. The difference is in the texture. Lotions are much lighter and less dense than cream, so they absorb more rapidly.

In Korea, those with normal or dry skin usually apply lotion before cream. However, if your skin is combination or oily, we recommend that you apply lotion as the final step of hydration, using it in place of cream. As it is light, it creates no sensation of heaviness and, unlike cream, it leaves no residue, so your skin will feel fresher. If you have dry skin or notice tightness as the season changes, apply lotion before cream for extra hydration.

—
METHOD OF USE
—

Applying lotion is one of the final steps in the Korean beauty routine. When you apply it depends on your skin type (see above).

How to apply a lotion:

01 Apply lotion after using serum and eye cream, and just before hydrating cream or sleeping packs. The trick is to put the lotion first in the palm of one hand, then to warm it a little by bringing your hands together.

02 Softly massage it into the face and neck, using light touches to facilitate absorption.

81

—
MYTH-BUSTING
—

'Because of its lighter texture, lotion is less effective than cream.' Wrong! We usually feel that liquid products don't give the same results as those with denser textures, but that is not the case. The effectiveness of a product is measured not by its texture, but by its formulation and the percentages of the ingredients it contains. This means that a cream can be very thick but contain fewer active ingredients than a lotion. The secret is knowing how to interpret the ingredients – those listed first are the major constituents – and use that information to purchase the products that are right for you.

## TIP

Do you have a dark make-up base? Mix it with lotion to lighten it. This will also make it much lighter in texture and more hydrating, while keeping the right tone.

## WHAT WE LIKE ABOUT LOTIONS

- ♥ THEY USUALLY COME IN BIGGER CONTAINERS THAN CREAMS, SO THEY LAST LONGER.
- ♥ THEY HAVE A LIGHTER TEXTURE AND ARE ABSORBED MORE EASILY.
- ♥ THEY ARE THE PERFECT ALTERNATIVE TO CREAMS IN SUMMER MONTHS OR IN VERY HUMID CLIMATES.

## OUR FAVOURITES

- ♥ *BIRCH JUICE HYDRO EMULSION* BY E NATURE.
- ♥ *ROSE ABSOLUTE VITAL FLUID* BY AROMATICA.
- ♥ *TEA TREE BALANCING EMULSION* BY AROMATICA.

## SUMMARY

LOTION OFFERS THE SAME BENEFITS AS A CREAM, HOWEVER THEY ARE MUCH LIGHTER, WHICH MAKES THEM THE PERFECT ACCOMPANIMENT FOR SKIN THAT DISLIKES THICK, GREASY TEXTURES.

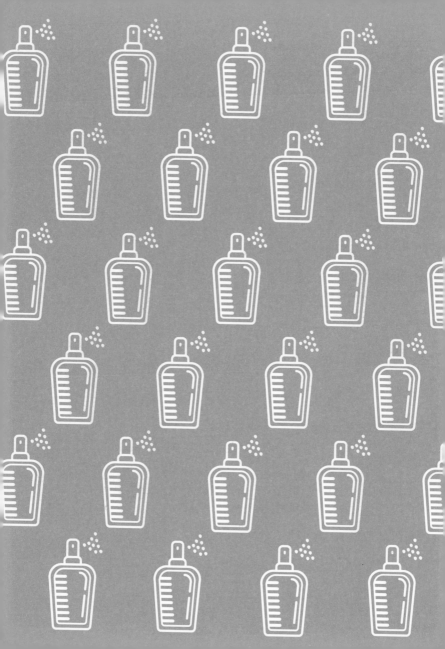

# CREAM
## 크림

**THE JEWEL OF K-BEAUTY.**

Even if you don't like cosmetics, you will certainly have a face cream in your beauty kit. And if you could take just one product to a desert island, it's highly likely that you would choose a cream.

### DESCRIPTION

Cream is the best of all moisturisers, having been used for centuries to treat and improve skin issues. There are many different types, and various ingredients have been tested to achieve the optimum results. Among cosmetics, cream offers the greatest variety of options in terms of texture, fragrance and presentation. It deserves its reputation as something special, something that makes us willing to spend more on it than any other cosmetic product.

It could be said that you can tell a person by their cream. After all, creams aren't chosen by accident. When you find the right one, you will fall in love with it, and if you have to change it later, you will be sad. You can probably remember the first cream that belonged to you, that no one else was allowed to touch, and that you used in tiny quantities so that it would last as long as possible.

—
METHOD OF USE
—

Applying cream is the final step of the Korean beauty routine, provided it hasn't been replaced by a lotion, and provided we don't include extra steps, such as applying sun cream during the day or a sleeping pack before bedtime.

We'll let you into a secret: the majority of creams can be used both day and night, as long as they have no sun protection factor.

However, a cream that you have enjoyed throughout your life can suddenly stop working for many reasons, the main one being changes in your skin. Like the rest of the body, your skin alters over time, and only by constantly checking in the mirror will you be able to tell if your favourite cream is still doing its job effectively. If the answer is no, it's time to find a better one.

How to apply a cream:

01 Apply cream as the final step of your beauty routine, before sun cream but after serum or lotion.

02 Always use a spatula if the cream does not have a pump, because placing your fingers in the container can transmit bacteria.

03 Spread cream from the middle of the face towards the sides, and from the chin to the forehead.

—

MYTH-BUSTING

—

'One cream for all ages.' If you read this somewhere, run, don't walk! In order for a cream to offer results, it has to have been formulated with top-quality ingredients which address the specific needs of the skin. Those needs change over time, and you mustn't over-stimulate it with things it doesn't require. For example, young skin does not need the level of hydration required by mature skin, so it would be a mistake for a teenager to use her grandma's moisturiser.

## WHAT WE LIKE ABOUT CREAMS

♥ THERE IS A GREAT VARIETY OF TEXTURES, FORMULAS AND FORMATS ON THE MARKET.

## OUR FAVOURITES

♥ *ROSE ABSOLUTE VITAL CREAM* BY AROMATICA.

♥ *MIDNIGHT BLUE CALMING CREAM* BY KLAIRS.

♥ *SNAIL BEE HIGH CONTENT STEAM CREAM* BY BENTON.

## SUMMARY

NO ROUTINE IS COMPLETE WITHOUT THE ESSENTIAL HYDRATION OF A CREAM.

## TIP

At night-time, add two small drops of oil (argan or marula, for example) to your cream in order to give extra nutrition to your skin.

# SUN CREAM
## 선크림

**THIS IS THE ULTIMATE SKINCARE
SECRET OF KOREAN WOMEN:
THEY PROTECT THEMSELVES
FROM THE SUN THROUGHOUT
THE YEAR.**

Sun is one of the principal causes of premature ageing, manifesting in such things as dark patches on the skin. The problem for many of us is that we only begin to think about sun protection when some of the ageing symptoms have already appeared.

There is one simple rule: always use sun cream before leaving the house, no matter if the weather is rainy, cloudy or cold, because the sun's rays will still reach your skin. Of course, using sun cream during the summer goes almost without saying, but remember to increase the SPF and apply the cream every two hours.

### DESCRIPTION

As the name suggests, sun cream protects the skin from the sun's rays. The most important part of sun cream is the filter, an ingredient, or group of ingredients, that works to stop the harmful effects of the sun on our skin.
Sun creams contain two different types of filters:

CHEMICAL FILTERS. Also known as organic filters, these seek to absorb or capture ultraviolet light and transform it into non-harmful energy. Among the most common are aminobenzoic acid, avobenzone, homosalate, octisalate, octinoxate and oxybenzone.

PHYSICAL OR MINERAL FILTERS. These block radiation by creating a reflective barrier. Creams that contain these will have titanium dioxide or zinc oxide listed in the ingredients.

—
METHOD OF USE
—

Sun cream is always the final step of the Korean beauty routine and must be applied shortly before leaving home in order for it to function correctly. It is applied after cream but doesn't replace it, unless the day cream contains solar protection.

How to apply a sun cream:

01 Apply sun cream after your hydrating cream or lotion.
02 Spread it from the middle of the face towards the sides, and from the chin to the forehead.

'Sun cream leaves my face white.' Physical filters usually do leave a white residue on the skin, but there are now many improved products on the market and their whitening effect is far less visible.

'I don't use sun cream because I have oily skin.' Sun creams used to be dense and greasy, and this gave rise to the false belief that they were unsuitable for oily skin. Nowadays, there are many good options for oily skin, including sun creams with light textures and oil-free formulations.

## WHAT WE LOVE ABOUT SUN CREAMS

♥ SUN CREAM FORMULAS HAVE EVOLVED TO THE POINT WHERE THEY ARE AS PLEASANT TO USE AS DAY CREAMS.

♥ THEY KEEP THE SKIN LOOKING YOUNG AND HEALTHY FOR LONGER.

♥ THEY ARE EVEN AVAILABLE AS SPRAYS, WHICH MAKES THEM EASY TO APPLY, SO THERE IS NO EXCUSE NOT TO USE THEM.

## OUR FAVOURITES

♥ *OH MY SUN PROTECTION MILK* BY YADAH.

♥ *I'M PURE CICA SUNCREAM* BY SUNTIQUE.

## SUMMARY

IF YOU DON'T WANT YOUR SKIN TO LOSE ELASTICITY, FIRMNESS AND CLARITY BEFORE ITS TIME, THE BEST THING TO DO IS APPLY A SUN CREAM EVERY DAY, REGARDLESS OF THE WEATHER.

# BB CREAM
## 비비크림/ 쿠션

**OFFERING HYDRATION WITH
COLOUR AND SUN PROTECTION,
THIS PRODUCT IS YOUR BEST
ANTI-AGEING SUPPORT WHEN
YOU'RE ON THE ROAD.**

Korean cosmetics owe most of their well-deserved fame to the quality of their BB (blemish balm) creams. Many years before they began to be fashionable in Europe, BB creams were already a basic product in the Korean daily beauty routine.

### DESCRIPTION

BB cream is a tinted day cream that includes a sun protection factor, and – like make-up – it can be blended over the skin to cover small imperfections and leave the complexion looking smooth and even. It's usually sold in tubes, often with applicators of varying sophistication. However, the BB revolution truly began when the creams began to be sold in cushion format.

Don't know what that is? Basically, it's a compact containing a damp cushion impregnated with the light tinted cream. What makes it so popular is that it provides all the benefits of liquid make-up in an easy-to-use form. The cushion allows you to apply just the right amount without wasting even one drop, and it provides great cover.

The BB compact is based on the same principle as the ink pads used with rubber stamps in post offices, but is far more sophisticated. Each cushion has up to 800,000 pores, which allow the make-up to filter in a uniform manner when pressure is applied. The cushion is made from a special material that can hold up to nine times its weight in water, so you get a decent amount of product for your money. Moreover, it is very hygienic.

Currently, many brands use the cushion format, either for make-up or BB creams. Cushions were launched in Korea in 2008 and keep on developing, so this is no passing fashion. Why choose a cushion? Because it's an easy and comfortable way to apply liquid make-up and dispenses the correct quantity of product. It sits on the skin in a very natural way and also provides good cover. It's also fantastic for travel, as the container is like a powder compact with application cushion and a mirror.

93

## METHOD OF USE

First, find the right shade for your skin tone. You should try BB cream on your jaw before making a purchase. Never try it on the wrist or the hand because the skin tone there is different from the face. BB cream is applied just like a make-up base, using fingers, a brush or a cushion applicator.

How to apply a cushion-format BB cream:

01 Press the cushion with the applicator disc until it absorbs a small quantity of the product.

02 Apply to the face with light touches, spreading it smoothly.

03 Repeat the process if you want more cover.

—

MYTH-BUSTING

—

'All BB creams are very white.' Well, yes. We know it's difficult to find a Korean BB cream that works well for non-Asian skin. Koreans have a very light complexion and the tones are designed for the local market. Fortunately, brands have seen that in order to build popularity in the Western market, they have to create a wider range of tones, so it is becoming easier to find a wider variety.

## WHAT WE LIKE ABOUT BB CREAMS

♥ THEY COVER SMALL IMPERFECTIONS WITHOUT LOOKING HEAVY, THUS OFFERING A MUCH MORE NATURAL APPEARANCE THAN A TRADITIONALLY THICKER MAKE-UP BASE.

♥ THEY ARE MULTI-FUNCTIONAL PRODUCTS, OFFERING NOT JUST HYDRATION, BUT SUN PROTECTION AND COLOUR TOO.

♥ THE CUSHION FORMAT IS EASY TO TAKE ANYWHERE AND CAN BE APPLIED HYGIENICALLY.

## OUR FAVOURITES

♥ *REAL FIT MOISTURE CUSHION* BY VILLAGE 11 FACTORY.

♥ *ILLUMINATING SUPPLE BLEMISH CREAM* BY KLAIRS.

♥ *UNICORN HEART LAKE CUSHION* BY MELOMELI.

## SUMMARY

BB CREAMS HAVE ALL THE PROPERTIES OF A DAY CREAM, THE BENEFITS OF A SUN CREAM AND THE FINISH OF A MAKE-UP BASE.

# SLEEPING PACK
슬리핑팩

**SLEEPING PACKS WORK WHILE
YOU SLEEP SO THAT YOU CAN
WAKE UP TO PERFECT SKIN.**

During the night, the skin is regenerated. Therefore, sleeping well and resting for a optimum number of hours means that you will wake up with brighter skin and more energy. Continued lack of sleep is reflected in our skin, not just our body: both will be dull, tired and lacking in vitality. While the natural nocturnal process of regeneration is absolutely essential, we can maximise the benefits by using sleeping packs.

DESCRIPTION

On the days when you use a sleeping mask – two or three times per week – it should be the last product in your daily routine, and can be used instead of hydrating cream. It comes in a jar and has a gel-like texture that is easy to spread over your prepared skin. It is not an unnecessary add-in to get you to spend more time and money on yourself. Sleeping packs usually contain powerful antioxidants that have regenerative properties. We especially love those with natural aromas, such as lavender, which help us to relax.

Fortunately, there is nothing complicated about using this product. It's applied just like a day cream, avoiding the eyes, and is removed with tepid water the next morning.

How to apply a sleeping pack:

01 Do the complete Korean beauty routine up to the last step. Apply the sleeping pack instead of the hydrating cream.
02 Spread it evenly over the face, neck and cleavage and massage in with small circles.

MYTH-BUSTING

'Sleeping packs stain and are sticky.' This is the most common excuse to avoid using this product in the daily routine, but it's incorrect. The sleeping pack formulations that we find on the market these days aren't sticky or uncomfortable, and they don't stain the pillow. While they can be greasier than some creams, the skin absorbs them all the same.

**TIP**
Use a silicon spatula
or brush to apply
your sleeping pack.

## WHAT WE LIKE ABOUT SLEEPING PACKS

♥   THEY ARE ONE OF THE EASIEST WAYS TO LOOK AFTER YOUR SKIN AS THE PRODUCT IS APPLIED AT BEDTIME AND LEFT TO WORK OVERNIGHT.

♥   SKIN IS MUCH SOFTER THE NEXT DAY. YOU DON'T HAVE TO WAIT WEEKS TO SEE THE RESULTS.

## OUR FAVOURITES

♥   *BIRCH JUICE HYDRO SLEEPING PACK* BY E NATURE.

♥   *FRESHLY JUICED VITAMIN E MASK* BY KLAIRS.

♥   *ULTRA NIGHT LEAF MASK* BY A. BY BOM.

## SUMMARY

SLEEPING PACKS GIVE YOUR SKIN ALL THE INGREDIENTS AND HYDRATION YOU NEED WHILE YOU SLEEP.

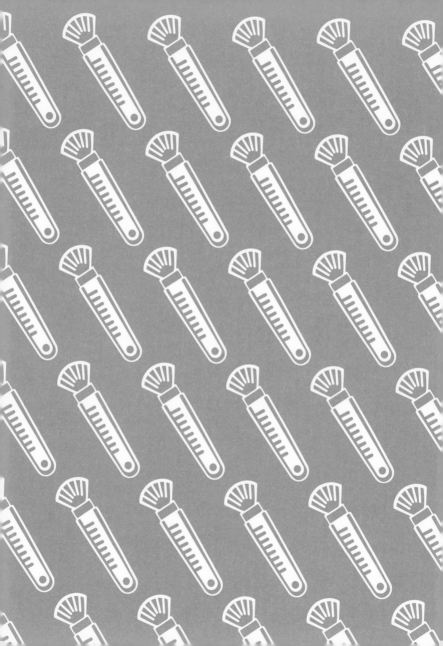

# 04

## THE KOREAN BEAUTY ROUTINE

한국의 스킨 케어

Now that you already know how Korean products work, it's time to let you know one of the best kept secrets of Korean cosmetics: the ten-step routine. Don't be surprised; it might seem strange, but once you understand it, you will see just how much sense it makes.

IT DOES INVOLVE A NUMBER OF DIFFERENT PRODUCTS, BUT SOME ARE USED ONLY OCCASIONALLY RATHER THAN DAILY: exfoliants, single-use masks, hydrogel patches and sleeping packs come into this category.

Perhaps you would prefer just one all-purpose cream? It doesn't exist, or if it did, it would be very expensive. The ten-step routine we are going to teach you will allow you to deal with all your skin concerns, from acne and dilated pores to dullness and wrinkles. Every step will help you to improve the appearance of your skin as long as you follow the complete routine in the purest Korean style.

THE ROUTINE MUST BE PERFORMED TWICE DAILY, MORNING AND NIGHT. Depending on the time of day, the steps vary slightly and some products can be replaced by others. The routine will also vary depending on the amount of time you have available.

# MORNING ROUTINE

---

**MORNING ROUTINE FOR BEGINNERS**

Everyone, no matter how expert, needs a basic routine. This applies whether you are just beginning or only have five minutes in the morning.

**01 CLEANSING** is the best thing you can do for your skin in the morning. Never skip this step.

**02 TONER** brings extra hydration to the skin. It prevents the feeling of dryness after cleansing and helps your cream to penetrate better. You can't do without it.

**03 CREAM OR LOTION** provides essential hydration. In fact, without it, there is no treatment, so this is always required.

**04 SUN CREAM** is needed every day, regardless of the weather. Never skip this step.

An expert routine requires two basic things: knowing your skin very well and having time to complete all the steps.

01 DOUBLE-CLEANSING is a two-step process that's always required, even though you may think you might already have clean skin after the previous night's routine. The fact is that after sleep, there are impurities, residues, dead cells and sebum to be eliminated. Also, this step helps to activate the circulation.

CLEANSING OIL removes all the products you have used the previous night.

WATER-BASED CLEANSER removes impurities and leaves the skin ready for the steps that follow.

02 EXFOLIANT, ideally a mechanical exfoliant, should be used whenever you can. It's best to use chemical exfoliants only at night.

03 TONER is essential to restore the skin's pH level after cleansing and to avoid the sensation of tightness.

04 ESSENCE will help the other products to penetrate better.

05 SERUM provides hydration with hyaluronic acid or collagen.

06 EYE CREAM or hydrogel patches help to decongest the eye area. They are great if you haven't slept much and notice your eyes look tired, or if you have bags under them.

07 LOTION AND CREAM are both applied and in this order if you have very dry skin. If your skin is normal, combination or oily, apply only one of these products.

08 SUN CREAM is the final step and can be applied as a cream or in a BB cushion format, which will also give a little colour to the face.

# NIGHT ROUTINE

---

The basic night routine is very similar to the basic morning one, but includes an extra step – the first cleanser. The skin accumulates toxins during the day, so keeping it clean is essential.

106

01 DOUBLE-CLEANSING involves two steps, and you have to do both, whether or not you're wearing make-up:

MAKE-UP REMOVER OR CLEANSING OIL must be used to remove make-up, any cream or sun cream and sebum from the skin. You can choose balm or oil format.

WATER-BASED CLEANSER removes impurities. Foams or gels are a good option.

02 TONER hydrates the skin after cleansing and prevents the feeling of tightness.

03 SERUM OR MASK Instead of applying sun cream, we can give extra care to the skin by applying a serum or a mask before the cream.

04 CREAM provides the final layer of hydration.

## NIGHT ROUTINE FOR EXPERTS

01 DOUBLE-CLEANSING is required, and is exactly the same as in the basic routine (see opposite page).

02 EXFOLIANT, specifically chemical exfoliant, is best used at night so that the skin will not be immediately exposed to the sun after using it. Remember, don't mix it with other AHAs or BHAs (see page 47), or with other physical exfoliants or enzymes. Exfoliant is not applied every day, so you can alternate it with other treatments that contain ingredients incompatible with it and thus avoid any risk of irritation.

03 CLEANSING MASK (peel-off clay) is also best used at night, when you generally have more time. Choose one that suits your skin type and include it in your routine once every seven to ten days. Clay masks absorb impurities and must go before any hydration step.

04 TONER is essential in any routine, but especially after using a cleansing mask because it re-balances the skin's pH.

05 SINGLE-USE FACE MASK is a hydrating treatment, but is not used every day, unless it contains ingredients that are non-aggressive to the skin, such as hyaluronic acid or collagen.

06 ESSENCE – although the face mask already contains essence, if you want to do the full routine, you have to apply it again after the mask. For this reason, we recommend that you remove any excess product from the mask with cotton wool or tissue and only leave on what your skin can absorb.

07 SERUM is best applied at night because it is a powerful treatment used for dealing with a specific issue.

08 EYE CREAM or hydrogel patches should be applied before face cream to create a protective barrier around the delicate eye area. Never use facial cream as eye cream. If using hydrogel patches, you can apply them at the same time as the single-use face mask, slipping them underneath it, to make the most of the 20 minutes.

09 CREAM is the best option at night, even though you might have replaced it with lotion in the morning routine. Cream is denser, but the texture won't bother you while you're asleep.

10 SLEEPING PACK replaces sun cream in the night routine, but does not have to be used every night. It provides an extra layer of hydration to the skin and leaves it looking perfect the next day.

108

**TIP**
If you forget the order of the steps, just check the density of the products. In general, you begin with the most liquid and end with the thickest. The sequence of applying products is known as layering.

# TRAVEL ROUTINE

Although I am now expert at the daily beauty routines, my work means I have to travel constantly, and I find it impossible to travel with everything I normally use. Below are some tips that help me to maintain my skin's condition when I'm away from home.

I START BY FILLING A WASHBAG WITH SAMPLES OF MY FAVOURITE PRODUCTS, the ones that always work and that I know I can combine without problems. If I don't have samples, I decant products into small bottles. Also, I take only one cream with me, even though I use various creams at home according to the appearance of my skin. The same goes for the rest of the products: I travel only with my favourites.

IF YOU HAVE TO DO WITHOUT ONE PRODUCT BECAUSE THERE'S NO SPACE, THAT WOULD BE EXFOLIANT. I don't use it daily; in fact, I can easily go up to ten days without using it.

FACIAL MISTS ARE PERFECT FOR KEEPING THE SKIN HYDRATED, especially when it is exposed to changes of environment, such as the dry air in an airplane. When travelling, we have to hydrate our skin more often, so I always include one in my washbag. The same goes for masks; you might even see me wearing one onboard! This way, I can avoid the sensation of dryness at the end of a flight.

# HOW TO BEGIN THE ROUTINE

If you have decided to incorporate the ten-step Korean routine into your skincare regime, you might be feeling a little overwhelmed at first, so here's some advice:

START LITTLE BY LITTLE. You don't have to start from zero but it is important to begin slowly, especially if you've never done anything like this before. In this way, you will understand which cosmetics offer most benefits and give the best results for your skin. If you don't know where to start, here's the answer: cleanser, cream and sun cream. If these three products aren't in your routine, don't experiment with others, such as essence.

FIRST PURCHASE? Opt for a good cleanser, as cleansing is fundamental. It might not be the most exciting product, but it's one of the most important because it's essential to apply subsequent products to clean skin.

KNOW YOUR SKIN TYPE. Korean cosmetics are almost always formulated for a specific skin type, so find out what yours is before you purchase anything. Even if you're told a cream is miraculous, it might not be the right one for you.

PREVENT RATHER THAN TREAT. Don't look for anti-ageing treatments if you don't yet have wrinkles; it's better to invest in a sun cream. Focus on what your skin needs and don't use treatments for problems you don't yet have.

LEARN ABOUT BRANDS AND THEIR PHILOSOPHY. You'll be using your cosmetics for a long time, so, just like any other products you consume daily, learn about the brand, the concept and the history that make it unique. Write a list of your favourite brands and everything you want from them, such as organic and vegan ingredients.

111

TIP
If you don't know where to start, begin with cleanser, cream and sun cream.

# 05

**NATURAL
INGREDIENTS IN
KOREAN BEAUTY**
한국 화장품에 사용하는 천연 성분

Without doubt, one of the most interesting aspects of Korean cosmetics is their composition because the ingredients they contain can be rather exotic. This chapter lists some of the most popular ones, and we think you're in for a few surprises!

## RICE EXTRACT

Also known by its scientific name, *Oryza sativa*, rice extract has antioxidant properties and both illuminates and softens the skin.

## BAMBOO

Thanks to its antioxidant, anti-inflammatory and hydrating properties, bamboo has been an essential ingredient of oriental medicine for centuries. Naturally, Korean cosmetics have incorporated it into their formulas.

## PEARL EXTRACT

Pearl extract is an authentic jewel for the skin. It can be used to give dull and tired skin an extra shot of clarity.

### SNAIL SLIME

This is the Holy Grail of Korean cosmetics. Snail farmers discovered that the slime produced by these creatures not only softened their hands, but also quickly healed small cuts and grazes. Its regenerative properties make snail slime a very desirable ingredient.

### GALACTOMYCES

Galacto-what? Fermented ingredients are very common in Korean cosmetics, and galactomyces (fermented yeast) is the most commonly used. It's a derivative of sake and considered one of the most effective ingredients in Korean cosmetics. It illuminates the face, tones the skin and regulates levels of sebum. It really does it all!

### CENTELLA

This small but powerful plant is one of the top ingredients at the time of writing, even though it has been used for centuries in Southeast Asian food. Its calming and healing properties are truly miraculous.

### BEE VENOM

Here's an ingredient with excellent anti-inflammatory properties. Who would have guessed? Known as natural botox, bee venom stimulates the production of collagen in the skin.

### BIRCH EXTRACT

The sap extracted from birch trees is used in a great variety of Korean skin treatments, and even replaces water in some products. This isn't just a passing trend as birch sap is very hydrating yet extremely light.

## ALOE VERA EXTRACT

Calming, regenerative and safe to use at any time (except just after sunbathing), aloe vera extract is a soothing gel and very popular although its soothing properties have been known about for decades. Aloe vera is also used in place of water in some products.

## PROPOLIS

Everyone's buzzing about it! Propolis is a mixture of resins that bees obtain from vegetable sources and use to seal their hives. It has antibacterial and antifungal properties, and also softens the skin.

## NATTO GUM

This fermented ingredient produced from soya is an excellent antioxidant and highlighter. If you've travelled in Asia, you have probably seen natto on restaurant menus, but be warned: fermented soya is an acquired taste!

## LIQUORICE

Thanks to its lightening and anti-inflammatory properties, liquorice root is a highly valued ingredient. Use it if your skin is dull, reddened, or has dark patches.

## TEA TREE OIL

Both antiseptic and antifungal, tea tree oil is one of the most ancient ingredients used in cosmetics. It offers many benefits to the skin, not least in soothing acne outbreaks. Indeed, dermatologists and scientists consider it as powerful as benzoyl peroxide, a medication often prescribed for acne.

## CHARCOAL

If you have oily skin or dilated pores, charcoal is the ingredient you need to incorporate into your routine, as it absorbs excess sebum and impurities. It's ideal for deep cleansing, and easy to find in masks and soaps.

## ALGAE

In recent years, the popularity of cosmetic products containing marine ingredients has increased because so many users have seen the benefits they provide. Algae is a group of aquatic plants that have been found to have regenerative and antioxidant properties. These are high in mineral salts, vitamins and oligo elements that are assimilated directly by skin cells and impart a much healthier and younger appearance.

## GINSENG

The secret of ginseng is in the root. It has many advantages when used in cosmetics: it is regenerative, helping the skin to recover elasticity, and is antioxidant (protects against the adverse effects of free radicals). It can be used at any age.

—
### WHITE TEA
—

Although lovely to drink, white tea is even better when applied to the skin because of its high polyphenol content. It's also an excellent anti-ageing ingredient, as it helps to produce elastin and collagen.

—
### CALENDULA
—

Sensitive skin always responds to this ingredient. Calendula has calming and repairing properties, and we recommend its use even on skin that has suffered years of exposure to the sun or that needs to heal.

—
### *SYN-AKE*
—

A synthetic form of snake venom, *Syn-Ake* improves skin elasticity and has a lifting effect, making it a powerful anti-ageing treatment.

—
### LOTUS FLOWER
—

An extraordinary cosmetic ingredient, lotus flower hydrates the skin, gives it clarity and even soothes the most sensitive skin.

# WHICH INGREDIENTS WILL SUIT YOUR SKIN?

The following information is arranged by skin type and lists the best ingredients for each one.

## OILY SKIN

If you have oily skin, you have probably used products containing salicylic acid, a derivative of aspirin. It has the effect of exfoliating the skin and cleansing pores deeply. Vitamin C also illuminates and evens the skin tone like no other ingredient.

Tea tree oil, a natural antiseptic and anti-inflammatory, is a fantastic ingredient for oily skin or acne. Witch hazel is also very effective at reducing spots, but THE TOP PRIZE GOES TO CENTELLA, WHICH CALMS IRRITATED SKIN, REDUCES ACNE SCARRING AND ELIMINATES EXCESS SEBUM.

If you haven't used this wonder ingredient yet, try a single-use face mask containing Asian centella and you will see what we mean. Of course, if you like using masks, those formulated with clay are excellent to combat oily skin and reduce pores.

Propolis helps to prevent acne outbreaks, thanks to its antibacterial properties. And if you have scarring, there's nothing better than snail slime for skin regeneration.

IT'S VERY IMPORTANT TO APPLY HYDRATING PRODUCTS TO OILY SKIN BECAUSE IF IT BECOMES DEHYDRATED, IT GENERATES EVEN MORE SEBUM. Use cosmetics with hyaluronic acid or niacinamide to keep your skin in good condition.

DRY SKIN

As dry skin is always desperate for hydration, HYALURONIC ACID WILL BE YOUR GO-TO PRODUCT. Squalene, a fatty acid that the skin produces naturally, is another ingredient that works miracles against dryness. We recommend vegetable squalene, which you will find in many masks and creams for your skin type.

121

Ceramides are naturally present in the skin, and their vegetable and synthetic versions are used in facials. They are perfect for re-establishing the skin's natural protective barrier. Two other popular ingredients used to treat dryness are honey and shea butter.

Even though dry skin doesn't require as much exfoliation as other types of skin, it is a good idea to exfoliate occasionally. In this case, use lactic acid, a very delicate option that won't damage the hydration barrier of the epidermis.

COMBINATION SKIN

USE INGREDIENTS FOR DRY SKIN ON YOUR CHEEKS AND OTHER DRY AREAS OF THE FACE, AND INGREDIENTS FOR OILY SKIN IN THE T-ZONE. This will help your skin look perfect.

## MATURE SKIN

USE BEE AND SNAKE VENOM TO STIMULATE THE SKIN TO PRODUCE ITS OWN COLLAGEN. This is more effective than directly applying products that contain collagen because most cosmetics don't penetrate the epidermis.

In order to exfoliate, use an AHA (see page 47), such as lactic or glycolic acid. Hyaluronic acid will help to keep your skin hydrated. Remember that hydration and ALWAYS USING SUN CREAM are the most effective ways of preserving a youthful complexion.

## SENSITIVE SKIN

Even if you have sensitive skin, we can recommend some products that will leave your skin as fresh as a cucumber!

CALENDULA, ALOE VERA AND CAMOMILE are three very delicate vegetable ingredients known for their soothing properties. Similarly, hyaluronic acid offers hydration without irritating the skin, so use it without fear.

Niacinamide works for sensitive skin (as long as it's not too concentrated), illuminating it and hydrating deeply. If you are a fan of natural ingredients, green tea and rice extracts are two very interesting options. When you choose a sun cream, opt for one with a physical rather than a chemical filter (see page 89).

# 06
—

**NATURAL**
**BEAUTY**
천연화장품

—

Natural facials are much more than a passing fashion: they are based on Korean philosophy and lifestyle. Like all natural cosmetic products, they are produced only with ingredients that are totally natural and effective.

At MiiN, one of our favourite brands is Aromatica, so we spoke with its founder, Jerry Kim, to learn more about the arrival of natural cosmetics in Korea. One of the many reasons we fell in love with this brand is because it's totally vegan and natural. We're sure you'll love it too! Here's what he told us:

*'IN 1997, WHEN I WAS STUDYING IN AUSTRALIA, I DISCOVERED THE FASCINATING WORLD OF AROMATHERAPY, WHICH IN KOREA AT THAT TIME WAS USED ONLY IN POPULAR MEDICINE. When I realised that the majority of cosmetic products contained artificial fragrances, I decided to create natural alternatives.*

*I began selling essential oils wholesale. I visited some of the most important brands in the cosmetics sector in Korea, but they weren't interested in natural ingredients. I came to the conclusion that if I wanted things to change, I would have to do it myself. I was aware that it wouldn't be easy to create a brand of natural cosmetics, but* I WAS CONVINCED IT WAS MY DUTY TO PRODUCE COSMETIC PRODUCTS THAT RESPECTED THE ENVIRONMENT. *Thus, Aromatica became the first Korean firm to apply aromatherapy to its cosmetics.*

*The name Aromatica comes from aromatherapy, which uses aromatic essential oils. Aromatherapy has only recently been applied to cosmetics; before that, the use of essential oils in skincare was limited to massage. The first cosmetic brands began to use essential oils less than 20 years ago.*

*In the beginning, it was difficult to enter the Korean market, as strong aromas were a new concept and many of our products were quite intense. For example, one of our successful products,* Rose Absolute First Serum, *originally contained three times the amount of rose oil that it does now. We had to adapt our formulas to the Korean market.*

128

*This serum is still our bestselling product because its rose fragrance is very popular. Nowadays, almost all brands have a line of rose-scented products, but they don't use pure oil. Instead they use rose water or extract, and they add artificial fragrances derived from petroleum.*

*Many young people love animals, so they appreciate that we are a vegan brand. Vegan cosmetic products are formulated with natural ingredients. As they don't use synthetic ingredients, they are safer for our skin and more respectful of the environment. They should not be confused with products that simply claim not to have been tested on animals.* VEGAN COSMETICS ARE NOT TESTED ON ANIMALS, BUT THE REAL DIFFERENCE IS THAT THEY NOT DO CONTAIN ANY INGREDIENTS OF ANIMAL ORIGIN.

*With regard to skincare, there are no magical routines; you just have to choose the right products for your skin type. After the age of 35 or 40, skin becomes drier, so it requires more hydration.*

*I have dry skin, so I wash my face with* Sea Daffodil Cleansing Mousse, *which is perfect for sensitive skin as it has less foam. Then I use* Sea Daffodil Aqua Toner *two or three times in a row to hydrate deeply. The next step is* Argan Intensive Hydrating Serum, *and I finish with* Jerry's Baby Hyalu Ato Cream *to hydrate. The* Jerry's Baby *line is hypoallergenic and contains no fragrance, so it's perfect for all ages.*

*It's important to share the message that our products are natural and organic, but we want our clients to truly appreciate the quality and the effectiveness of our cosmetics.'*

JERRY KIM
FOUNDER OF AROMATICA

# 07

—

## K-BEAUTY
## DO'S AND DON'TS

절대 안 되는것들

—

## APPLY COSMETICS IN THE CORRECT ORDER

In the Korean beauty routine, the order of application makes a difference to the result. In general, we start by applying the most liquid products before moving on to those with a denser texture. However, while texture is important, function is even more so. For example, there might not be that much difference in density between a toner and an essence – it all depends on their formula. In this case, follow the recommended order (toner before essence) so that you achieve the desired results. Toner works to balance the skin's pH after cleansing and must be applied before any other hydrating product or treatment.

## REMEMBER TO CARE FOR YOUR NECK

Use the same day cream on your neck that you use on your face. Just like facial skin, neck skin loses elasticity, firmness and hydration over the years.

### DON'T USE ANTI-AGEING PRODUCTS TOO EARLY

Of course we all know that prevention is important, but getting into anti-ageing products too soon can be counterproductive. Cosmetics with anti-ageing properties contain ingredients that young skin doesn't require. For prevention, it is more useful to keep the skin hydrated from a young age. There is no exact age at which to begin using anti-ageing products; it depends on your genetic inheritance and lifestyle. The answer should be found in the mirror: look at your skin rather than marketing hype.

### HYDRATE YOUR SKIN CONSISTENTLY, NOT JUST WHEN IT APPEARS DRY

Our skin sends us signals, and dryness can be one of them. Lack of hydration leads to flaking. If you see this symptom, it means that you have not hydrated your skin enough. Be on the lookout for changes like this and take action. Of course, the best preventative measure is to act before the signs appear.

### DON'T FORGET THAT EVEN OILY SKIN NEEDS HYDRATION

Many people don't hydrate their oily skin because they are taken in by the myth that using cream on the face will only increase production of sebum. In fact, it's quite the opposite. Oily skin must be hydrated to avoid excess production of sebum, which is generated in response to a lack of hydration. The secret lies in knowing how to choose a cream that hydrates the skin yet isn't heavy and doesn't leave residue. Gels are best for oily skin.

—
USE SUN CREAM ALL YEAR ROUND, NOT JUST IN THE SUMMER MONTHS
—

By this point in the book, you know how bad it is to neglect sun protection. Skin has its own memory, and all the sun exposure that you have accumulated during your life will appear sooner or later in the form of dark patches or premature lines and wrinkles. WHATEVER THE WEATHER, ALWAYS USE SUN CREAM.

—
DON'T USE JUST MAKE-UP REMOVER AT NIGHT
—

It's so easy just to slap on some make-up remover before going to bed, but it really isn't the best option for cleansing the skin. It takes only an extra minute to do this step correctly and remove make-up with the double-cleansing method. Your skin will thank you for the rest of your life.

—
REMEMBER TO DOUBLE-CLEANSE, EVEN IF YOU'RE NOT WEARING MAKE-UP
—

We've already told you: it takes only a minute more to clean the skin properly, and the difference is significant. Even if you're not wearing make-up, your skin will have been exposed to dirt or pollution. The first step of double-cleansing, using a cleansing oil, removes any oil from the skin. The second step, a water-based cleanser, removes impurities.

## DON'T RUB PRODUCTS INTO THE SKIN TOO ROUGHLY

Rubbing vigorously won't make the skin cleaner. It will just cause irritation and redness. There is a method for applying liquid products that is much more beneficial to your skin: pour a small quantity of product into the palm of one hand and warm it by placing the other hand over it. Next, gently press both palms all over the surface of the face.

## AVOID USING MECHANICAL EXFOLIANTS IF YOU HAVE SENSITIVE SKIN OR ACNE

Exfoliants work to clean the skin deeply, but if you have very sensitive skin or acne, you must avoid mechanical exfoliants. They contain solid particles that will scratch and irritate the skin, making it easier to spread infection.

136

## DON'T THINK 'MISSING ONE DAY WON'T MAKE A DIFFERENCE'

As in most areas of life, a consistent approach produces the best results. If you suddenly stop a treatment, you won't achieve the same desired effects.

—

## DON'T COMBINE INCOMPATIBLE INGREDIENTS

—

There are some ingredients that cause a reaction if used together. Read the list of ingredients carefully, or seek advice from your pharmacist or a beauty expert on the products you are using in your skincare routine and ask if they are compatible.

—

## DON'T WISH FOR MIRACLES

—

Cosmetics work on the surface, so they can achieve improvements, but these will never be magical. Using cosmetics is better for the health and appearance of your skin, but you must always be aware of what you can achieve.

—

## KEEP PRODUCTS IN THE RIGHT PLACE

—

137

Heat, light, humidity...all of these factors can adversely affect the composition of cosmetic products. For example, vitamin C oxidises when exposed to light and will lose its effectiveness. Similarly, high temperatures can cause products to deteriorate. Read the recommended storage advice on the packaging and find an appropriate place to keep your products so that they maintain their properties.

—
### DON'T FORGET TO CHECK YOUR PRODUCTS' EXPIRY DATES
—

Just like food, cosmetics have an expiry date, which must always be taken seriously. Generally, the product container indicates how long their properties can be maintained once they are opened. It's best to note when you began using a product so that you don't forget this date.

—
### DON'T SHARE YOUR PRODUCTS – OR USE ANYONE ELSE'S
—

It's all too easy to dip into your mum's cream, your sister's cream, your girlfriend's cream, but not all products work for all skin types. Cosmetics are something very individual because not everyone has the same needs. For this reason (and for hygiene's sake), it's important to personalise your skincare routine.

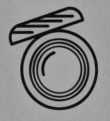

# 08

---

## KOREAN
## BEAUTY TRENDS
한국의 트렌드

---

# MAKE-UP

Koreans have a well-defined style of make-up, quite different from what we're used to seeing in the West, and the complete opposite of American make-up trends. IN KOREA, THE OBJECTIVE IS A NATURAL APPEARANCE. It's not about using make-up, but rather about using products that give the skin a perfect and nude finish.

FACE

In Korea, people generally use BB creams with different functions and degrees of cover, blending them over the skin to achieve an even tone and hide imperfections. The objective is to give skin a healthy and dewy appearance, so products with extra hydration and highlighting properties are sought after. For a perfect finish, we recommend a subtle highlighter and a hint of blusher on the cheeks.

**Look for products with extra hydration and illuminating properties for a dewy appearance.**

In the West, foundation is used more than BB creams, although BB creams are becoming more popular. The coverage of foundation is usually heavier, giving the complexion a totally uniform tone and hiding open pores (there are even specific primers for this). In general, a matte finish is desirable, so some form of powder tends to be used over the make-up base. In Korea, we look for the famous glow effect.

The techniques of contouring, once used only by professionals or created at home just for special occasions, have become more commonplace. Today many people use contouring on a daily basis. It's the same with highlighter, which gives a touch of light to casual make-up and contrasts with the matte finish on the rest of the face.

Blusher tends to be more coloured in the West, where we use a variety of tones. In Korea, the most popular colours are peach and soft rose.

EYEBROWS

KOREAN MAKE-UP KEEPS EYEBROWS BASICALLY STRAIGHT AND MADE UP IN A NATURAL WAY. We only fill in the eyebrow to emphasise the natural shape. However, micropigmentation (cosmetic tattooing) is very popular. In Western make-up, the eyebrows are usually arched and heavier, with less intense colour in the area above the tear duct, and thinner towards the outer eye.

In order to give a natural, enlarged eye effect, Korean beauty uses pearly eyeshadow with gloss, always in quite soft tones (pinks, corals and earth shades). Eyeliner or a dark eyeshadow, more often brown than black, follows the natural line of the eye without adding a flick at the end. It's a soft line intended to define the eyelashes in a very subtle way.

ASIAN EYES HAVE A ZONE KNOWN AS *AEGYO SAL* (ADORABLE CHARM). This is the area just underneath the lower line of eyelashes, where some people have natural bags that are nothing to do with tiredness. These are believed to give a much younger appearance to the face. Indeed, in recent years it has become popular to have cosmetic surgery to accentuate them. In Korea, the bags are highlighted with pencil or pale eyeshadow, and can even be drawn on or made more pronounced by tracing the lower line with a very light touch of a darker shade.

145

The eyelashes of Korean women aren't very long or thick, so curlers, mascara and even false eyelashes are commonly used to increase their density.

In the West, eyes tend to be very heavily made up, using various colours according to the season. Bright colours and a wide range of matte tones are often used on the upper eyelid and under the lower line of the eye. It is also common to use pronounced eyeliner to create the look known as 'cat eyes'. This has the effect of enlarging the eyes and gives greater intensity to the make-up. In Korea, the trend is more towards 'puppy eyes', making the eyes appear rounder to give the melancholic expression of puppies and is associated with a more youthful appearance.

## LIPS

Korean women like to use shaded lip colour. This involves applying a greater intensity of colour in the centre of the lips and a lighter colour at the edges, which gives a very natural, fresh and appealing effect. As you might expect, Western lip make-up is much more pronounced. In recent years, matte lipstick has become popular, and the look is intense, with the same density of colour all over the lips. For those who are more daring, there are also metallic lipsticks in shades such as blue, green and grey.

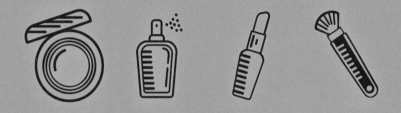

# BASIC KOREAN
# MAKE-UP ROUTINE

### 01

After completing your facial cleansing routine, end with a moisturising cream or lotion, and you can then even the skin tone with your usual BB cream. Remember that BB creams usually have a sun protection factor (SPF), but if you use another type of product for this first step, it is very important to apply one containing an SPF after the moisturising cream. Once you have applied the BB cream, you have two options: if you really like the luminous finish of Asian women, simply leave the BB cream to set before going on to the next step. If, on the other hand, you have a tendency towards shininess, you can use some translucent or sebo-regulating powder to avoid this. If you choose the second option, don't make your make-up base too matte. The main objective is to look dewy and healthy. Luminous skin is beautiful and youthful.

### 02

Outline your eyebrows with a specific colouring pencil as close as possible to your natural tone. Although Koreans prefer a straight brow, you don't have to follow their example. Simply define the natural shape of the eyebrow and fill it in gently, using a small brush to blend the colour so that it isn't too harsh.

### 03

Once the eyebrows are ready, choose an eyeshadow (cream, powder or pencil) in a soft tone to apply to the upper eyelid. As the aim is to create a natural effect, you can apply it directly with your finger or use the applicator if you prefer. It should be blended so that there is no sharp difference with the lower part of the eyebrow.

**04**

Use a fine brush and a dark brown eyeshadow to define the shape of the eye. Start by drawing a line as close as possible to the eyelashes, judging the length according to the shape of your eye. Asian women tend to avoid the tear duct and begin about two-thirds of the way along. They finish at the outer end of the eye without making a flick. Once you have drawn the line, blend it slightly with a brush for a more natural finish. To give greater luminosity to your eyes, you can apply a lighter shade of eyeshadow and a gloss one either above or below the tear duct.

**05**

Choose a blusher in a shade of coral or soft rose. Using a brush, apply the colour softly in the area of the cheekbones and blend it a little towards the temples. Use the same method to apply cream or cushion-format blusher.

**06**

If your eyelashes are straight, curl them a little with the help of a curler before applying mascara. If you are fortunate enough to already have curly eyelashes, just apply your mascara and move on to the next step.

**07**

Now apply your favourite lipstick or lip gloss to the centre of your upper and lower lips. Use your finger to blend the colour outwards, being careful to keep the colour most intense in the centre, with the lighter tone towards the outer corners of your mouth. This will give a pretty shaded effect. If you want your lips to appear dewier, you can apply lip balm as a preliminary step. This will also keep your lips hydrated for longer.

# SKIN COMPLEXION

In recent years, not only have new products arrived from Korea, but we have also seen many new trends and fashions in the world of beauty. At MiiN we take an interest in everything. The trends change according to skin type, but they are worth examining because the outcome can be surprising.

## DEWY SKIN

If you follow all the trends from Korea, you will certainly have heard the term 'dewy' in reference to the appearance of skin. This is how Korean women want their skin to look, unlike women in the West, who want their skin to look matte. Take note, though: dewiness has nothing to do with oiliness. The shine on Korean skin is not the result of excess sebum. It is a luminous quality that suggests health.

## HONEY SKIN

This goes one step beyond dewy skin. If someone tells you that you have skin like honey, it's a compliment because it means your skin is beautiful.

Try to imagine a jar of honey. How would you describe it? Its colour is even, transparent, radiant and shiny. This is how your skin should look with the right facial routine. There are some tricks to achieve this: facial oils help, as they nourish the skin deeply, maintain hydration and give a plumping effect.

## GLASS SKIN

As with honey skin, it is also a compliment to tell someone they have glass skin. In this case the look is flawless and translucent, like a crystal.

We already know that Korean women care about the appearance of their skin, but it is intriguing that they would go so far as to try to have skin like crystal. And do you know what is even more surprising? They never stop trying!

They are always seeking perfect skin: moist, free of imperfections, clear and transparent like crystal, with no artifice and no make-up. Their skin is like an immaculate sheet or canvas where the artist begins work.

How do they achieve this? There is no magic product that gives the desired finish in one hit. The key is constancy in following the Korean skincare routine (see chapter 4, page 101), applying layers of products to hydrate the complexion as much as possible, and always using the right products for their particular skin type. However, here are some tips to help you achieve the crystal effect:

01 After cleansing, softly exfoliate the skin.
02 Apply an essence or serum with a light texture, and use hydrating ingredients, such as hyaluronic acid.

In order to achieve glass skin, we recommend using products with very liquid textures. After a few days of following the complete routine, the result can easily be seen after applying serum, when the skin is in an optimum state of hydration.

152

—

## CLOUDLESS SKIN

—

Cloudless skin takes us beyond the surface; it is a trend that works with our ideal lifestyle. It encourages us to be respectful of ourselves, our body and our environment, taking care of our skin but also being aware of all the external factors that can damage it.

Like a clear sky on a sunny day, cloudless skin has a healthy appearance with no distractions. Unlike other trends, it is based more on health than appearance, so the final result is only part of the process.

Any other reasons for the name? Well, stressed skin has a cloudy or dull appearance and we are looking for the opposite of this. The stress hormone cortisol makes the skin more vulnerable and reactive, so it is more easily irritated. Asian centella (see page 116) is one of the best ingredients to calm the skin.

We can only achieve cloudless skin if we care for ourselves inside and out. We need to eat well, avoid exposure to free radicals, control our stress levels and get enough sleep. Taking these steps will help to protect us from external threats to our skin and prevent premature ageing – signs of which include inflammation, hypersensitivity, acne and dark patches.

We have to monitor our skin and decipher the signals it sends to keeping it looking its best – cloudless!

153

01 TIRED SKIN – to avoid, try to sleep between seven and nine hours a night, and maximise the cellular renewal that goes on during that time by applying intensive treatments such as sleeping packs.

02 DARK PATCHES are caused by excessive exposure to the sun's ultraviolet rays on a daily basis. As soon as the patches appear, see your dermatologist and look for cosmetics that contain arbutin, vitamin C or liquorice extract, which have anti-inflammatory and lightening effects. Also, choose skin products and sun cream that have a high sun protection factor and use them every day.

**03 OPAQUE SKIN** without shine is a sign of stress. Try to dedicate a few minutes daily to unwinding; your skin and your body will thank you. There is nothing better that reclining on the sofa wearing a soothing face mask.

**04 DEEP LINES** indicate a lack of elasticity, which can be caused by the action of free radicals. Did you know that if you hydrate the skin deeply, it's less susceptible to free radicals? Hydrate, hydrate, hydrate.

**05 BLOCKED PORES** are associated with contamination. Cleansing and exfoliation are two fundamental steps of the routine that help to eliminate all type of impurities and dirt.

—
*7 SKIN METHOD*
—

Just when we think we know everything about the Korean routine, a new method of toner application appears. We are always being surprised! Note: this process might seem like a joke but it isn't at all. Korean women really do it and it works!

The *7 Skin Method* consists of applying toner seven times. Yes, that's right: seven times. Seven layers of toner on your skin. Why? To hydrate it and leave the skin radiant (not oily). The method is very simple and you don't need any new products, just your toner.

**01** Clean the skin.
**02** Dampen a couple of cotton wool pads with toner and dab them over the skin, or pat the toner onto your skin directly using the palms of your hands.
**03** Allow the toner to absorb.
**04** Repeat steps 2 and 3 six more times.

The *7 Skin Method* is a shock treatment for all types of skin that are dehydrated or lack clarity. It's ideal after prolonged exposure to the sun, or during travel, especially long flights. In fact, it's great at any time when the skin has been subjected to change, such as climate or stress. This method is much more effective than using a day cream because it is water-based and penetrates the skin more easily.

—
*JAMSU*
—

What is one thing that you never do after putting on make-up? It's probably safe to say that you don't immerse your face in a bucket of water, do you? Korean women, of course, are different. Their technique for keeping the skin soft and matte after applying make-up is called *jamsu*, which means 'submerge in water'.

*Jamsu* is very easy to do: simply apply your BB cream, cover it with a generous application of matte powder, then...submerge your face in a bucket of cold water for 30 seconds. You then pat the face dry with a towel or a cloth, no rubbing, just light touches or a little pressure to absorb the dampness from the skin. After that, you apply the rest of your make-up: eyes, cheeks, lips and so on.

This technique ensures that make-up remains intact for much longer, and reduces the appearance of shine during the day. However, it doesn't work with every skin type. We recommend it only for oily skin during the summer months; doing it in cold weather could dry the skin too much.

—

—

The average refrigerator often contains one of the best skin cleansers, but it's only recently come to our attention. The magic product is carbonated water. Korean women have discovered all the benefits it has for the skin, and already made it an alternative to other facial cleansers.

Carbonated water provides mini-exfoliation for sensitive skin. Having bubbles, rather than the solid particles found in some exfoliants, it doesn't irritate the skin so much. It's therefore ideal for combination and acne-prone skin because it helps to control the production of sebum and removes excess oil from the skin. It also has strengthening properties and encourages clarity. Another advantage of carbonated water is that it contains less calcium than tap water. Do be sure to use plain carbonated water, not fizzy drinks.

We recommend doing this twice a week, even if you have oily skin, and you can do it at any time of day, although it's more effective at night.

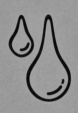

# 09

---

**KOREAN
SKINCARE
ANSWERS**
자주 묻는 질문들

---

You may have some questions as you take your first steps into the world of Korean cosmetics. As the sector is in constant evolution, even experts (with skin as lovely as actresses in K-dramas) suffer moments of confusion.

## HOW MUCH TIME SHOULD I DEDICATE TO DAILY BEAUTY ROUTINES?

The minimum is 5 or 10 minutes in the morning, and 20 minutes at night. It is an effort, but once you start to see the changes, it will become easier day-by-day. Even if your life is frenetic, you should see the time spent doing the routine as your chance for relaxation and pampering. The routine can last up to 50 minutes or an hour, depending on the number of steps you do. For example, it can take longer if you are doing your weekly exfoliation or a specific treatment because some masks require 30 minutes.

—
HOW MUCH TIME SHOULD I WAIT BEFORE DOING THE NEXT STEP IN
THE ROUTINE?
—

You only have to wait a few seconds between applying each product.
However, this does depend on your skin type and which step you're
doing. If your skin is oily, it probably takes longer to absorb products,
but it's still just a matter of seconds, so don't worry. In the case of
toner or essence, it's possible to go on to the next step before the
skin has absorbed them completely, and doing so actually directs
the active ingredients more efficiently.

—
AT WHAT AGE DO KOREAN GIRLS BEGIN TO LOOK AFTER THEIR SKIN?
—

In Korea, girls begin to look after their skin from an early age,
having observed their mothers. Also, it is easy for them to access
suitable cosmetic products because some brands focus on a young
or even very young market. The use of cosmetics in K-dramas and
the influence of celebrities have also contributed to lowering the
age when girls begin to use cosmetic treatments. Many brands now
target consumers in their twenties rather than their forties.

—
WHICH KOREAN COSMETICS HAVE HAD THE GREATEST SUCCESS WITH
WESTERN CONSUMERS?
—

Without doubt, masks are one of the star products. Those now being
launched by some Western brands bear no comparison with the
great variety of Korean products. BB creams are also popular among
Westerners, but not in comparison with their scale of popularity
in Korea.

—

—

South Korea's most important contributions to the world of cosmetics are their innovative formulas, the unique design of their containers and the fact that it's fun to use their products. Many US and European brands have conquered the global market with conventional products, but it's been a long time since consumers have seen anything new, and that's why Korea is now coming to the fore. Korean cosmetics represent an adventure in terms of their content, texture, application and design. Consumers were looking for something new and Korean cosmetics have met their needs.

—

WHY HAVE KOREAN COSMETICS ACHIEVED SO MUCH WORLDWIDE SUCCESS
IN THE PAST TWO YEARS?
—

This question has been comprehensively answered by the PR department of Wishcompany Global, a firm located in South Korea, whose commercial brand is Klairs:

*'Korean cosmetics are known in the global marketplace for their high quality, innovative formulations and reasonable price. The Korean cosmetics market is full of very good brands and quality products. This is because the Korean cosmetic industry is very competitive and has developed and created not only new brands and products, but also many consumers through the power of the internet.*

*Consumers of Korean cosmetics include groups aged from 10 to 40, who are also very active online. Through social media, people can communicate with anyone, in any place and at any time, and express almost anything.*

*So, what would happen if Korean products weren't good quality, if their price was too high without justification? Only the brands that offer quality can survive the constant judgement of social media. Thus, the true power of brands lies online, not just in South Korea, but throughout the global market.*

*Klairs is a good example of success. Not only has it survived, it has thrived because it has become a top brand that now has more than one and a half million fans worldwide, outside South Korea. Klairs has created its own communication platforms and publishes informative digital content that is also fun. It communicates directly with clients and shares its brand philosophy: "simple but enough". This focus has been appreciated by millions of people and helped to position the brand very well on the principal global social media platforms.'*

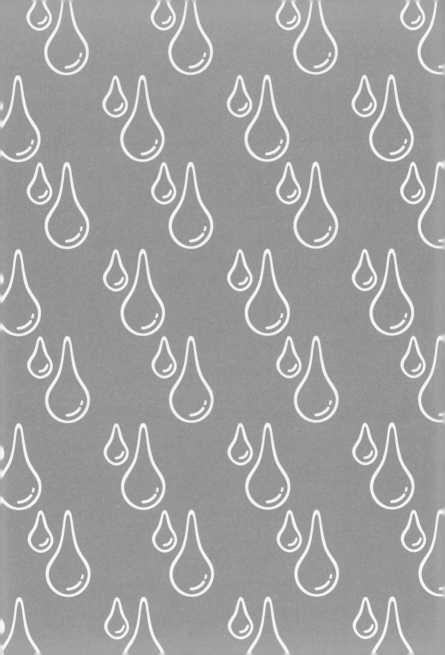

# 10
—
## KOREAN SKINCARE TIPS FOR MEN
남성 화장품

—

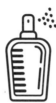

ACCORDING TO THE MARKET RESEARCH COMPANY EUROMONITOR, KOREAN MEN USE MORE SKINCARE PRODUCTS THAN MEN ELSEWHERE IN THE WORLD. Indeed, their per capita spending is four times greater than the second group in the list: the Danes.

The male skincare sector turns over $1 billion a year in South Korea, and is expected to grow by almost 50 per cent in the next five years. Korean men don't just buy aftershave and day cream. There is more and more demand for anti-ageing products, masks and facial mists.

Two of the founders and directors of our favourite brands are men: Jerry Kim of Aromatica (also see pages 127–129) and Soungho Park of Wishcompany (Klairs). They have spoken to us about their experience with male skincare products, both as consumers and businessmen. Over the following pages, they share their impressions with us.

# THE VISION OF JERRY KIM

FOUNDER AND DIRECTOR OF AROMATICA

HOW DO MEN IN SOUTH KOREA LOOK AFTER THEIR SKIN? DOES IT DIFFER FROM THE REST OF THE WORLD?

'There is no substantial difference between Korean and Western skincare, but in South Korea we don't generally use products or deodorants with very intense fragrances. We are more interested in the properties of a treatment than other aspects such as smell.

In our daily routine, Korean men normally use a cleanser, a toner and a hydrating lotion. If we want to add a product for a more complete routine, we apply an exfoliant, or products that increase clarity or offer anti-ageing properties. In South Korea, men are interested in skincare and spend a lot of money on cosmetics, which has encouraged international brands like Lab Series, SK-II Men and ULOS to try new products for the male market in South Korea before launching in other countries.'

'The basic routine includes cleanser, toner and hydration. We wash our face with tepid water and next we apply a foam cleanser. Due to excessive production of sebum, men's skin tends to be a little oilier than women's, but it's important to avoid aggressive soaps, as they can irritate and dry the skin. I recommend cleansing foams, such as Aromatica's Tea Tree Balancing Foaming Cleanser, a soft cleanser formulated with organic aloe vera and tea tree oil. After cleansing, we apply toner and hydration.'

DO MEN USE THE SAME PRODUCTS AND STEPS AS WOMEN IN THEIR ROUTINE?

'In 2016, the turnover of the male beauty sector in South Korea was approximately $1.2 million, with an increase of 10 per cent every year because of growing interest from men. According to Olive Young, the biggest health and beauty shop in Korea, personal care sales have increased by 40 per cent every year from 2014 to 2016, and the new trend is that men, like women, pay attention to small details. They're no longer interested just in basic products; they also look for specific treatments, either to control pores and sebum, or to cover imperfections with coloured products, such as BB creams.

Many men take an interest in the functions and the results offered by the products. They want clearer skin and to delay the signs of ageing, as well as treatments for acne. Currently, the majority of men only use basic products for skincare, but we anticipate an increase in the number of men purchasing diverse and varied cosmetics, just as women do.'

—

—

'I have light and very delicate skin, so even as a teenager, when the production of sebum was at its greatest, I had to use a lotion with hydrating properties. Some people think that I have clean skin and small pores for my age, but I have to hydrate my skin daily as it tends to form wrinkles.

172

I use only Aromatica products for skincare. I begin my routine by washing my face with Sea Daffodil Cleansing Mousse. Next I shave with a shaving cream. Before using water to clean my face, I use Sea Daffodil Aqua Toner twice again and apply Argan Intensive Hydrating Serum. Next I use Calendula Juicy Cream for an extra touch of hydration. Before going out, I finish my routine with the Natural Tinted Sun Cover Cushion because it contains SPF and evens my skin tone.'

—

—

'As the male beauty market increases, brands are launching exclusive male skincare lines. Olive Young sells more than 20 brands of male skincare with all kinds of products: toners, lotions, essences, peelings, *anti-ageing treatments, exfoliants, eye creams and treatments for hyperpigmentation. Of course, there are also many unisex products on the market, such as single-use masks, clay masks and BB creams.'*

# THE VISION OF SOUNGHO PARK

FOUNDER AND DIRECTOR GENERAL OF WISHCOMPANY

HOW DO KOREAN MEN LOOK AFTER THEIR SKIN? IS THERE ANY DIFFERENCE BETWEEN SKINCARE IN SOUTH KOREA AND IN THE REST OF THE WORLD?

*'South Korea has the most important cosmetics market in the world. Men are very interested in their appearance, which is why they purchase this type of product. There are two types of client. The first group is interested in skincare, and the products and routine are similar to women's (not including make-up). The steps are: cleansing, toner, essence (or serum), cream and sun cream. They*

also use BB cream. The second group is interested in personal care, and many brands cater for this market, offering a wide range of all-in-one products. The skincare routine of people in this group is more basic: a single product containing toner, serum and cream, plus a sun cream.'

'There are fewer steps in the male skincare routine, though it doesn't differ much from women's. Men don't normally use make-up, so can skip some steps, such as make-up remover.'

IN THE KOREAN MARKET, IS THERE A GOOD VARIETY OF SPECIFIC PRODUCTS FOR MEN OR ARE THERE MORE UNISEX OPTIONS?

'Some clients use unisex products, while others prefer lines exclusively for men. The fact is that brands are constantly introducing new products, some of them male make-up products, like BB creams or cushions.'

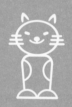

# 11
—
## KOREAN
## BEAUTY
## TRAVEL TIPS
한국 여행 팁
—

If you visit South Korea, it's worth allowing at least three days to go shopping in Seoul. Cosmetics shops are among the city's principal attractions, but there's much more to see and do. You'll probably return to Seoul because you've fallen in love with one of the hundreds of cafés, or because you want to fill your suitcase with clothes and gadgets.

# COSMETICS
# AND BEAUTY

Let's start with what we're most interested in: cosmetics. Where can we purchase all the latest K-beauty products? THE VERY BEST AREA FOR BEAUTY SHOPPING IS MYEONG-DONG. This area is very touristy, but if your passion is cosmetics, you can't miss it. Prepare yourself for an onslaught of shops, promotions and people, but all your favourite brands, and the best-known ones, have their shops in this famous street. You will need at least three hours to walk the entire length of it and to take everything in. Don't forget to keep a list of all the products you want. Even if you don't purchase anything, you'll leave loaded with samples!

THE MORE COMMERCIAL BRANDS SOMETIMES HAVE SEVERAL SHOPS JUST A FEW YARDS APART, so if you don't find a product in one, just walk a little further along and try the next branch you come across.

This area is full of great places to eat, so you can snack between shops or have dinner after shopping. And if you're a fan of Line cosmetics, you can't leave Myeong-dong without visiting their flagship shop and taking a photo with the adorable Brown, a huge teddy bear at the entrance.

ANOTHER AREA WHERE YOU WILL FIND ALL THE COSMETICS YOU WANT AND MORE IS GANGNAM. There are lots of shops in the streets around the famous station. You might have to queue to enter some of them, such as the Kakao Friends flagship store, but we promise it's worth it.

Both Gangnam and Myeong-dong have multibrand beauty shops, such as Aritaum and Olive Young. All the products that have reached Europe started in these shops. With a little luck you can find yourself holding the next Korean cosmetic success months before it becomes an essential product in Europe.

If you're looking for something trendier, don't miss Cree'mare and its great variety of brands. It offers many products that aren't made in South Korea, so you can discover which Western cosmetics the Koreans like the most. Chicor is another multibrand shop with a similar concept. It doesn't have the most commercial brands, but tries to stock the very best – small brands with a special philosophy that makes them unique. Many of our favourite products have come from here.

181

Still in the beauty world, why don't you leave shopping behind and try a pampering experience? Skincare is an art in South Korea, so beauty salons must be luxurious. If you want to try the best, don't leave Seoul without visiting A. by BOM, a very special place where you will find all the beauty services you desire: hairdressing, manicures and make-up salons. It's become an essential destination for celebrities.

Of course, manicures are a very important ritual in South Korea. There are specialists who will turn your nails into true works of art. Indeed, the designs at Unistella are worthy of the catwalk. You can't return home without getting a manicure as they are unforgettable.

OUR FINAL PIECE OF BEAUTY ADVICE IS TO ENJOY SOME TIME AT A SPA. You deserve it after a 12-hour flight! You can visit one of the famous Korean *jimjilbang* (spas), but if you want to feel like a princess, make an appointment at any of the three Shangpree spas in Seoul. They have more than 20 years of experience and you will be in the hands of experts.

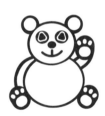

# EXPERT TIPS

FOR RETURNING HOME WITH THE BEST COSMETICS

Check out the dates when limited editions are released. Most brands launch exclusive editions in collaboration with other brands, and these products are even better than normal. Follow the official social media accounts of your favourite brands so you don't miss anything.

Follow beauty vloggers to keep up with the latest trends. They are usually on top of all the latest developments and can provide useful information about products before you commit to purchasing them.

When you know what product you want, keep a photo of it on your phone. You will then be able to show the products in shops to the staff who will then know exactly what you are looking for.

There are so many cosmetics shops close together that it's worth browsing all of them before making a purchase. The offers can vary even within the same brand's range.

It's normal to receive samples or free products when you make a purchase. If this doesn't happen automatically, don't be afraid to ask.

# FOOD AND DRINK ESSENTIALS

Even though we love cosmetics, every time that we're in Seoul we like to discover new places that have nothing to do with beauty. Korean fashion, gastronomy and culture have so much to offer, and the streets of Seoul have many fascinating and unusual corners to explore.

Typical Korean dishes are easy to find almost anywhere in the city. We recommend *bibimbap*, a tasty mix of rice, tender minced meat, vegetables and eggs; *tteokbokki*, fried rice pastries with fish and spring onion; *kimchi*, fermented Chinese cabbage, a superfood found on every Korean dining table; and *jjajangmyeon*, noodles in black bean sauce with pork, soy sauce and vegetables.

Barbecued food is very typical of South Korea. It's easy to find places that offer this type of food, but ask for recommendations. A famous dish is black pork from the island of Jeju (a place also known for producing many cosmetic ingredients). A good place to try this is Black Pig Seoul, very close to the COEX shopping mall.

Seoul does have vegan options, but they can be difficult to find. The best thing to do is to download the HappyCow app, which shows places with vegan and vegetarian options close to where you are. Some of our favourites are Plant Café, Yummyomil, Huggers and Loving Hut.

Ikseon-dong, close to Jongno, is a district of the capital that's really taking off. Here you can find many typical restaurants and cafés in traditional Korean homes that have been restored. It's not very touristy, and some of the streets are only for pedestrians. It's a peaceful neighbourhood with small shops run by young entrepreneurs. The atmosphere is modern, yet traditional – a real experience.

The cafés in Seoul are the perfect places to enjoy people-watching and local life. There are so many that it would be impossible to try all of them in one visit. For this reason, we've made a small selection for you:

SEOUL COFFEE: This stylish café is located in Ikseon-dong, a very popular area with locals, which already says a lot. What we like most is the combination of traditional and modern. You can truly enjoy Korean style and design. The menu is also unique, not at all conventional. In recent years, the trend in South Korea has been for European-style places, which were seen as chic and trendy. However, this is changing, and greater value is being placed on Korean culture, which is seen as modern and elegant. That's why places like Seoul Coffee are so fashionable. *www.seoulcoffee.kr*

CAFÉ MENON: If we had a café at MiiN, this is what it would look like. Located in the Mapo-gu district in Hongdae, it is cute and pink, with cosmetic products on the second floor. What's not to like? Note: you must try the puddings.

MAJESTEA: A tranquil space with spectacular views, this café in Cheongdam-dong is the perfect place to enjoy good tea in the Gangnam district.

ORIOLE: Not so much a café, more a place to have a drink and enjoy views over the entire city. It's worth visiting both day and night, as the panorama is stunning and the atmosphere is very romantic. Oriole is in Hae-bangchon, close to Itawon.

# DID YOU KNOW
# THAT IN KOREA...

...The first mass-produced make-up was launched in 1910.

...Beans were used as a cleansing soap after mixing make-up and water, as they contain saponin, an effective cleansing agent.

...Lotions were made from juice extracted from plants such as pumpkin stems.

...Rice and millet were used as make-up, after mixing with water or oil, so that they could stick to the skin.

...Apricot and peach oils were used to treat liver pain and helped to hide freckles.

...Safflower oil, rich in vitamin E and essential fatty acids, is used to increase the skin's natural moisture and shine.

...It's typical to eat with metal toothpicks at traditional Korean barbeques, as wooden toothpicks are flammable.

...There are two different ways of saying goodbye in the Korean language, depending on if you are leaving or the person you are speaking with is leaving.

...It has one of the highest rates of cosmetic surgery operations in the world.

# EPILOGUE

We very much hope that you will want to try some Korean cosmetics now that you've finished reading this book. We have really enjoyed introducing you to them and hope we have eased you into this fascinating subject. Start gradually, and remember that we at MiiN were once beginners too!

K-beauty is much more than a skincare routine; it's a lifestyle that will change not only your appearance, but also how you feel about yourself. Millions of people all over the world have found their perfect skincare routine with Korean cosmetics because Koreans know the importance of the smallest details.

There is a specific facial routine for every skin type and we want to help you find the one that's right for you. Remember that we're here to answer any questions as you step into this marvellous world. See you at MiiN. We await you with open arms!

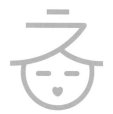